'Another book worthy of reading. Andrew Pike condenses, in a brilliant manner, complex and often confusing subjects of intention and sensations. He guides the reader through the quiet, deeper, inner sense of self that a of rampant speed and unrelenting bom disturbances.'

T0173657

– David Berceli, PhD, CEO of Trauma ...
Tension and Trauma Releasing Exercises (TRE)

'Although Andy Pike's new book is entitled, *Intention and Non-Doing in Therapeutic Bodywork*, I believe the work deserves a much wider, more general audience. For *Intention and Non-Doing in Therapeutic Bodywork* is a blueprint, complete with a large number of immediately practical exercises, for how to be a better human being, more present, more often, and less reactive in the process. Recommended.'

– *Kit Laughlin, M. Litt., founder of Stretch Therapy and author of*
Overcome Neck & Back Pain

'This deeply inquiring work invites the therapist to value not only the acutely subtle world of touch, but to self-inquire into the unseen yet palpable inner presence needed to bring an underlying truth and wholeness to the work between therapist and client. A beautiful, insightful masterpiece and guide for anyone working in a body-based therapeutic environment.'

– *Janet McGeever, co-author of* Tantric Sex and Menopause:
Practices for Spiritual and Sexual Renewal

'It is unusual to come across a mind that can delve so deeply into such an ethereal subject while simultaneously insisting on the embodiment of the truths discovered. You will feel Andy's insight throughout this book. His inspiring words, delicate descriptions and creative metaphors are alive, as is the essence they carry.'

– *Dr Graham Mead, MD, creator of the InnerSense Program*

'In this book Andy skilfully takes us into the detailed and nuanced world of sensation-based awareness, leading readers to greater richness, clarity and efficacy in their work. This text is a tremendous gift to astute bodyworkers who recognize the limitations of technique-based work and are ready to explore deeper states of therapeutic insight.'

– *Ryan Hallford, RCST, host of* The Craniosacral Podcast
and internationally accredited BCST instructor

of related interest

Touch is Really Strange
Steve Haines
Illustrated by Sophie Standing
ISBN 978 1 78775 710 3
eISBN 978 1 78775 711 0
...is Really Strange series

Cranial Intelligence
A Practical Guide to Biodynamic Craniosacral Therapy
Ged Sumner and Steve Haines
ISBN 978 1 84819 028 3
eISBN 978 0 85701 012 4

Yoga and Science in Pain Care
Treating the Person in Pain
Edited by Neil Pearson, Shelly Prosko and Marlysa Sullivan
Foreword by Timothy McCall
ISBN 978 1 84819 397 0
eISBN 978 0 85701 354 5

Intention and Non-Doing in Therapeutic Bodywork

Andrew James Pike

Foreword by Ged Sumner

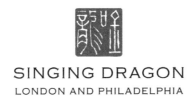

SINGING DRAGON
LONDON AND PHILADELPHIA

First published in Great Britain in 2022 by Singing Dragon,
an imprint of Jessica Kingsley Publishers
An Hachette Company

1

Copyright © Andrew James Pike 2022
Foreword copyright © Ged Sumner 2022

A CIP catalogue record for this title is available from the
British Library and the Library of Congress

ISBN 978 1 78775 898 8
eISBN 978 1 78775 899 5

Printed and bound in Great Britain by CPI Group

Jessica Kingsley Publishers' policy is to use papers that are natural,
renewable and recyclable products and made from wood grown in
sustainable forests. The logging and manufacturing processes are expected
to conform to the environmental regulations of the country of origin.

Jessica Kingsley Publishers
Carmelite House
50 Victoria Embankment
London EC4Y 0DZ

www.singingdragon.com

Contents

List of Figures

List of Experiential and Hands-On Exercises

Foreword

Andy has brought together many strands of wisdom in this book. What particularly stands out is the in-depth description of space and stillness. It is the ongoing theme of the book. It is refreshing to read about it as I don't often see it talked about or written about in the world today. This book takes you on a voyage of discovery of ancient wisdom from eastern yoga and meditational practices and more recent wisdom from an amazing bodywork therapy that investigates space and presence through touch.

Exciting pieces include some wonderful quotes, a whole series of felt-sense awareness exercises that define intention and non-doing while figuring out what that generates in the mind and body. I'm not sure that anyone has defined intention in such detail. Andy explores tendencies, impressions and sensations that arise in the body and mind as a result of intention and doing. Andy looks at the idea of original nature and finding a deep state of dynamic stillness at the same time as exploring trauma states that arise in the body and mind from unresolved experiences.

Really, the book is about finding embodied non-doing and generating a repose that is not seeking, judging, or generating an agenda. This is the essence of biodynamic craniosacral therapy and many spiritual traditions. Andy has derived a unique science in what he calls Cranioga, an intriguing blend of yoga and craniosacral therapy that gives people a change to deepen into their systems and appreciate the nuance of their body and mind.

Andy's background of Vipassana meditation, physiotherapy, bio-dynamic craniosacral therapy and yoga come through in the book as a synthesised wisdom that all body therapists, yoga practitioners and meditators should consult.

Ged Sumner
Director of Body Intelligence

Acknowledgements

This book was conceived and compiled due to my being inspired and influenced by a number of outstanding people over a few decades:

Notably the eloquent Dr Graham Mead, my spiritual brother. Throughout all the years I have known him he has always met me by surrendering to the importance of being present, whatever the circumstance.

Tao master Ged Sumner, who caught my attention from day one with his ability to share the insight of embodied non-doing in a contemporary manner, unburdened by superstition or dogma.

A number of honourable Zen teachers who spared time to share insight with me in years gone by, namely: Venerable Myokyo-ni, Martin Goodson, Rev. Master Daishin Morgan, Glenn Wallis Roshi, Ross Bolleter Roshi, Arthur Wells Roshi, Mary Jaksch Roshi and Amala-Sensei.

S.N. Goenkaji, whose wise words and kind smile conveyed deep insight and compassion. The Vipassana meditation environments he pioneered, established and developed have cultivated global insight, benefiting many people.

My graciously accepting mother and father, who have always given me free rein to follow the yearning of my heart, despite the unconventional nature which it often presented.

My son Luke, who has plunged into the deepend of this journey with little prompting and has given me confidence that his generation have a potential zeal for dancing with the profundity outlined in the content of this book.

Also thanks to Asuka Shiroshita-San, a fellow forest dweller, who shared many words describing the intricate nuances of nature, which in many cases I presumed were too subtle to be labelled.

Thank you to Di Harris for her diligent work with reformatting some of the images and for her skill and passion in her work.

And finally, thanks to everyone I have encountered who has been willing to share the insight of TI/ME passing. In those moments, we are in love – we are 'This'!

Preface

The igniting spark for this book took place a couple of decades ago when I realized that I was operating, like many bodywork therapists, by dedicating and applying skills without resting in the source of my own being. At this time, I discovered that bodywork therapists, especially those 'working' with the body, are in a unique position to experientially understand the nature of their own presence, while treating, and are potentially able to share this presence free from intention or expectation. The felt-sense understanding of treating in this way is as subtle as it is intense, and will be referred to throughout this book as 'insight'. Insight can be talked about and intellectualized forever and a day, but cannot truly be understood unless there is a tangible awareness of the arising and passing nature of body sensations alongside the realization that they are inseparably related to one's own reactive tendencies, impressions, memories and expectations. It is this sensation-based awareness which puts bodywork therapists in a capable position to glean deep insight during and following each treatment they provide.

Years later, following this realization, I combined what I had opened to with the content of a manual I was writing for the postgraduate Body Intelligence trainings on intention and non-doing. That is when the form of this book took shape.

Lack of insight can result in the subtler body expressions being veiled to the therapist, creating reliance on mechanical or esoteric techniques to assist a client's well-being. Such approaches will always be tacitly lacking something, but it is hard to ascertain what it is that is missing. This book, therefore, has been written for bodywork therapists who wish to increase both the understanding and efficacy of their treatments, while enabling the treatment sessions they provide to become a catalyst for resource and insight, both for themselves and their clients.

This subject matter can, at times, appear complex and perhaps even labyrinthine. At these points, it is useful to refer to the associated awareness exercises, to help experience what is written, rather than letting the intellect override what the words are pointing at.

The topic of intention and non-doing requires a number of metaphors and allegories to entice the reader to sidestep recalcitrant patterns of abstract thinking, as well as to support the mind into realizing its own inherent limits. Again, if confusion persists, it will be helpful to return to the experiential exercises to glean a more tangible felt-sense understanding.

There is space beneath each of the experiential exercise subcategories for the reader to pencil in noteworthy insights to refer to and reflect on.

The complex mind wants to read what is already familiar and known, because the mind regards what is perceived as familiar as simple. However, non-dual simplicity (felt-sense insight) reveals itself only when the 'known' ceases to obscure it. So, try to persevere with any intellectual confusion; indeed, let it culminate as a palatable intensity which has the capacity to dissolve the limitations formed by the accrual of the past (known). This does not mean that this book is encouraging a therapist to forget their accumulated knowledge, but rather to abandon being controlled by it. Awareness of such subconscious control dissolving is, in and of itself, insight. Such insight lends a whole new way of relating to imminent phenomena by accessing non-abstract noumena, i.e. that which cannot be understood by mere words. It is proposed that this insight is invaluable for bodywork therapists to realize and 'non-doingly' apply in their practice.

The majority of chapters are focused on the importance of the therapist's awareness and understanding of their own surreptitious identification to body sensations and their relationship to reactive tendencies, impressions, memory fluctuations, expectations and resulting intentions. This is the realm which needs to be explored to truly understand non-doing. Chapters 11 and 12 cover the understanding of the client's intentions and reactive habits and how to help the client access and apply a process which empowers them in the direction of embodiment, health and eventually 'engaged non-doing' (END), i.e. wakeful non-reactive wholistic contact to themselves and others – the end of subconscious doing.

There are annotations throughout the book which refer the reader to the endnotes in order to help describe and expand on deeper aspects in a given sentence. Many words are also provided with quotation marks to illustrate the potential ambivalence a particular word could evoke, if taken out of context. In addition, there are a large number of acronyms used to save repeating words too often, and these are referenced in the glossary.

The book contains words and terminology from many countries around the world to help convey and expand meaning. These will be displayed in italics and expanded on in the glossary. It is of course useful to obtain understanding by reading contemporary words and phrases in one's own commonly used language wherever possible, but, occasionally, ancient words from different languages hold deeper meaning compared to languages such as English. This is especially true when a particular word condenses a whole English sentence (or in some cases a whole paragraph) and highlights the need for felt-sense understanding rather than relying on verbose intellect. Such words can provide greater felt-sense intimacy to their deeper meaning, especially when relating them to the cultural context they derive from. So, the words in the glossary have been chosen for their ability to condense many aspects of the thesis introduced in this book.

Interestingly, some cultures have put particular emphasis on trying to explain certain subtleties which have been relevant to the culture over many centuries, and sometimes millennia. For example, the Japanese language has a large array of different words that describe the subtle sensations and/or sounds in the body just prior to the vitalizing emptiness free from thought (*mushin*). It is hard to find such words in other languages, although there are words describing different subtleties in other languages, which may be unique on account of their evolving alongside a particular cultural history.

There are probably many languages which offer many other words that could help deepen our understanding of intention and non-doing. Nevertheless, the languages used in this book are the ones I have been most exposed to, so they are the ones I feel most confident with in regard to their meaning, and even then there are probably differing translations to some of the words.

I apologize in advance if the contents of this book offend or conflict with any beliefs you may currently have. My hope is that this this book will encourage the reader to inquire experientially and go beyond beliefs, rather than deny or extinguish them.

The layout of this book may at times appear a bit disjointed. The reason for this is because the fundamental theory of a topic like this needs to be touched upon and then blended into experiential understanding. With this experiential insight it is expanded upon with both theory and insight combined. The felt-sense insight will help open the ability to understand deeper seemingly paradoxical theory, which in turn will open to deeper insight. There is a richness to this approach, as the theory will become alive and this aliveness, not the theory itself, will then act as a key to open the unknown. That way the 'hard problem of consciousness' is no longer stuck in a bias theory loop. In other words, the known is no longer hindering the simplicity of realizing 'This'.

It might also be useful to note that this book is not intending to promote a protocol or technique for bodywork therapists. As mentioned, the hope is that it will inspire the therapist to inquire into the source of her or his being. Such inquiry enhances the volition to help others which reciprocally helps oneself. If, as the reader of this book, you find yourself sufficiently intrigued, or if something seems to ring as a truth within you, then please take this further by reading Appendix 3. It is here you will find a way to take the priming information of this book into a place where you can continue to deepen and develop your insight into something very profound and liberating.

Having said that, Chapter 12 details an effective therapeutic process which I have developed over the years. I have included this to serve as an example for when and how access attention and non-doing can percolate into bodywork therapy sessions. But please note that access attention and non-doing can be included as an ally to any bodywork methods.

A note on the 'access' experiential exercises detailed in this book: some people will resonate with particular body regions more than other regions. It is good to be mindful of this inherent propensity and to investigate what works best for you. Be a pioneer of your own felt-sense discovery – it can open up a whole new way of perceiving.

So, summarizing and expanding on the preface: this book is dedicated to those who wish to understand more about the essence of body-based therapies and the deeper reasons for the beneficial effects they can have. Moreover, this book is for you to glean insight of embodied non-doing, which is a felt-sense understanding that does not rely on mere intellect.

Both orthodox and alternative therapies place much emphasis on the intentional use of techniques which attempt to alter this or that. Yet, health expresses itself optimally in an embodied relational field free from intention. This book will, therefore, be looking at how we, as therapists, skilfully navigate between intention, attention and non-doing while treating clients. The non-doing aspect is especially interesting, yet very often misunderstood, in that it is far from being a form of passive resignation. Understanding and being with the non-doing aspect of this navigation is the essence of effective safe touch and opens up a relational field free from psychological habits and restraints. So, in order to become clear about non-doing, it is essential to first understand what is meant by intention (doing), be aware of it, and not 'do' anything to add to it or change it. This is a form of yielding to 'what is', whereby the presence of engaged non-doing is a catalyst for enabling vitalized change and the expression of health. To be with this presence, rather than intentionally trying to change something based on past impressions or future projections, can be a huge relief to the physiology both in one's own body and in others'.

In the context of a therapeutic setting, intention is affected by a therapist's past exposure to life, which is then modified in the present and projected to help manifest a desired future outcome. As a result, such projection will always be influenced by, and identified with, an accumulation of tendencies, impressions, fluctuating memories and expectations[1] (TI/ME). As such, intention is bound by TI/ME, both as far as this acronym goes and literally with regard to our relative association with chronologic time. Consequentially, intention can hinder the expression of health, despite the limited positive mechanical effects attained via intention-driven techniques. That said, intention is profoundly useful when it is used to promote attention. Intentional attention to help uncover the undercurrent of subtle sensations can be the key to open an awareness of the whole with insight. This will be explained throughout this book.

Engaged non-doing is, therefore, the outcome of 'seeing' things in a unique way without reacting to the past or future. It is primed by a practice of intentional attention, which, ironically, leads to the dissolution of intention. It also leads to the felt-sense awareness of subtle sensations as they arise and pass away. By noticing the transitory nature of these sensations, without reacting to them, the contents of thought (TI/ME[2]) dissolve, enabling non-dual health to optimally express itself.

'By embodying non-doing, the cycle of TI/ME is undone and health gets to express itself.' (END therapist's interpretation of *wu wei*)

Chapter 1

Wholistic Awareness

You are not a drop in the ocean.
You are the entire ocean in a drop.

RUMI

1.1 Beyond the dot

One day, a tutor, seasoned in the art of therapeutic non-doing, entered the classroom and asked a group of students to prepare for a surprise written test. They all waited eagerly at their treatment tables for the exam to begin. The tutor handed out the exam papers with the text facing down. Once they had all been handed out, the students were asked to turn over the papers. To everyone's surprise, there were no questions – just a black dot in the centre of the sheet of paper.

The tutor, seeing the expression on everyone's faces, told them the following: 'I want you to write about what you see.' The students, perplexed, got started on the inexplicable task. At the end of the class, the tutor received all the exam papers and started reading each one of them out loud, in front of the students.

All of them, without exception, defined the black dot, trying to explain its position in the centre of the sheet, the hue of its blackness and size of its circumference. After they had all been read, the classroom was silent and the tutor started to explain: 'I'm not going to mark you on this, I just wanted to help you reorientate your way of perceiving. No one wrote about the white part of the paper. Everyone focused on the black dot – and this is the same thing that can happen when we, as bodywork therapists, treat people. We have a whole piece of paper which is ready to be acknowledged, but our tendency to focus on the particular leads us to perceiving only isolated fragments, rather than the whole. This perspective impels us, as therapists, to try and alter or join the fragments. Yet, it is this very intention that prevents us from meeting the wholistic nature of the client.'

More often than not our life is based on a dualistic interpretation of what we perceive. Yet, if we only focus on the discernible size, shape and colour of the dot (interpretation and accumulation[1] of sensory input), then we can ignore the bigger understanding and miss appreciating the potent quality of the paper on which the impression of the dot is highlighted. A therapist's simultaneous awareness of both the dot and the paper is akin to their felt-sense awareness hovering 'between' phenomena and no-thing. In other words, being intimately involved with the entire interpreted spectrum of perceived objects (phenomena) as well as the entirety of non-duality. Non-dual insight is appreciation that the essence of phenomena and noumena[2] are not different, they are just relative and absolute presentations of awareness.

The paper/dot allegory is used here to set the scene and help illustrate how therapists can fall prey to the habit of being over-focused. Too often we get caught in trying to change what is perceived, rather than encouraging a quality of wholistic perception, which unveils the ever-changing expression of nature itself.

◆ EXPERIENTIAL EXERCISE 1

The dot and beyond
Pratyahara

Figure 1.1: Dot expressing space

◆ With a black pen, draw a round dot on a blank piece of white paper.

◆ While sitting comfortably, place the piece of paper at arms length in front of you, or on the floor.

◆ Look at the dot without giving in to distractions for two minutes. Then close the eyes.

◆ Try to keep the eyes closed.

◆ We are dissociating from the sense of vision here, not to negate it in the long run, but to realize how this sense has become reactive to objects. These objects form a distractive association in the mind, preventing our awareness from perceiving the changing nature of our sensations and thoughts. So, for now, keep the eyes closed.

◆ Notice the impression of the negative image of the dot (which will either be white or some other lightish colour) in the mind's eye.

◆ Try to sustain this image.

◆ The mind is like a naughty child. To begin with it does the opposite of what you want it to do. If you shut out the other distracting impressions, the mind will automatically make the nature of the distracting impressions more intense.

◆ So, persevere with the awareness of the dot's impression in the mind.

◆ Just as important, notice the absence of the dot when it has eventually dissolved. This is the equivalent of the white paper in the dot and paper story.

◆ Notice this absence for a few minutes and then gently open the eyes.

◆ What quality of body sensations do you feel after this exercise?

1.2 The movie

Let us now expand on this understanding by using as a metaphor the event of watching a movie. If we were to start watching an enthralling film, on a television, the unfolding story would draw us in and we would, unwittingly, start to identify with the characters in the film. This is the hallmark of a good film and a big reason for our wanting to watch it. In other words, we lose ourselves in it. We even see the background in the movie as a three-dimensional landscape. But when we walk up to the television and touch the picture, we notice that it is actually just a screen.[3]

So, it is interesting to realize that, despite part of us being lured into the unfolding film, the screen itself, through which all the pixels of illumination are seen to be changing, does not change. It remains exactly the same throughout the duration of the movie. The characters and scenes are merely distortions of light which we evaluate and identify with. The reality is that the film is a light show which stimulates our conditioned and identifying habits. However, when we lose our identification to the unfolding movie, and we are aware of its absence, we can perceive the actual reality of a screen relaying a dynamic show of light.

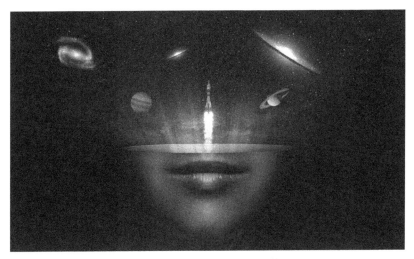

Figure 1.2: The universe unveiled

We all have the capacity to notice the screen while watching a movie.

Similarly, we all have the capacity to notice the stillness with which we are endowed. As therapists, when we realize this at the felt-sense level, within ourselves, it enhances a relational field with another. A relational field of this nature provides a client's system with the optimal opportunity to recuperate and reorganize.

CLINICAL NOTE

Both our body and our mind are endowed with the potential of expressing our original nature (dynamic stillness), in each and every moment of our lives – all we need is to perceptually awaken to this reality.

Yet, one cannot wake up if the state of 'sleep' is taken for being awake.[4]

In the clinic, therefore, we need to set the scene to enable ourselves, and our clients, to perceive the 'characters, light and screen' for what they really are.

In order to set this scene, it is useful to encourage the aware-ness of three inherent qualities in and surrounding both the client's body and our own body: safety, space and stillness.

Chapter 2

Feeling Safe

*No man ever steps in the same river twice, for it is not
the same river and he's not the same man.*

HERACLITUS

2.1 Setting the scene to notice the screen

As bodywork therapists, our training and practice put emphasis on the art and science of touch enabling another to find enough safety in their body for it to express health. The word 'safe'[1] can conjure an image of a person in hiding, secure from potential danger,[2] like diamonds in a vault being protected from the threat of being stolen (feeling safe – perspective one). Or, it could be interpreted as feeling immune to danger, free to function at an optimal capacity with the pliant adaptability of a flowing stream (feeling safe – perspective two).

The first perspective focuses on the threat and being free from it, whereas the second perspective pertains to the feeling of being okay despite potential disruption and, eventually, benefiting from it. This is also known as being safely embodied or anti-fragile.[3]

Being embodied with the feeling of being safe, therefore, is not the same as being defended, or even being resilient, like a shield or a rock (respectively), which obviously has its place if there is a tangible physical threat. It is more like the steady unagitated nature of a gentle flowing stream, with its ability to accommodate[4] and move beyond restrictions. This kind of fearless fluidity can seem paradoxical to the intellect, because while its adaptable nature flows with life, its essence comes from a deep and resourcing stillness. This is much like the secure resourcing a young child receives when her or his caregiver is available, supportive and implicitly able to communicate a fearlessness from their loving attention and calm presence.

If we 'safely' prevent a client's inquiry into the patterns of experience in their inner world, then the safety we provide will be a form of resistance, thereby perpetuating the need to feel protected, which becomes a never-ending cycle. Therefore, as therapists, we provide a sensitive and secure contact which resembles the contact a child requires to grow and explore. Yet, we do not prevent the client from learning and adapting to circumstance, and, at some point, entering the ocean of independence (see Appendix 2).

A client requires the ability to fluidly adapt in the face of circumstance in order to optimize their exploration and expression in the world, much like a developing child.[5] Such fluid versatility is a key quality inherent within the autonomic nervous system.[6] As one's awareness of this physiologic capacity increases, reactivity to stimulus decreases, i.e. the observer and the observed become more and more intimate as equanimity presides. When a client is guided/reminded of their fluid adaptability, their awareness starts to interface with an aspect of their being which cannot be analysed (*savikalpa*), but can be felt (*nirvikalpa*). This is our original nature.

So, as engaged non-doing (END[7]) therapists, we actually encourage the felt-sense awareness of the 'bigger picture' by providing a non-intentional felt-sense reference for the client – we embody the insight of the ocean for the client to gravitate towards, without pulling them into it.

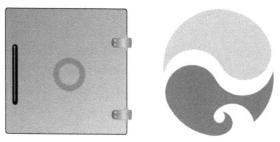

Figure 2.1: Vault safety and fluid safety

The autonomic nervous system (ANS) is 'trained', by experience, to react in a number of different ways. These could be reactions mimicking fragility or escaping (as mentioned), or a rigidly resilient manner (like a rock). Interestingly, the ANS isn't necessarily at the mercy of experience; when someone is embodied (explained later), then pliant adaptation can replace reactivity. The type of reaction or pliancy will correspond to how the ANS functions and relates to the world. Therefore, when the client's mind is not able to accommodate sensory input with adequate equanimity, the felt-sense of their body will likely be more vulnerable to dissociative tendencies and feeling fragmented. The mind does not give up the felt-sense of wholeness for fun. It is utilized as a strategy[8] to function in the face of overwhelm.

The therapist is there to help a client gather themselves together and gradually perceive more wholeness, allowing them to soften into the sense of safety.[9] Yet by far the most valuable contribution the therapist provides is to 'allow' the increasingly fluid nature of the client to be touched in a way that reflects the potent insight of their original nature, which is an invaluable resource in that it helps one begin to benefit from disorder rather than being destroyed by it.

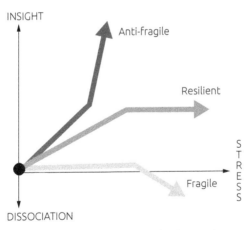

Figure 2.2: Anti-fragile/fragile graph

Therefore, an appropriate environment and a specific kind of therapeutic touch serve as a verification for inherent safety, especially when a client's system is overwhelmed.

Nevertheless, if this reference becomes relied on, and the client never discovers their own inherent resource, then such fluid-like safety will be limited, due to dependence on the environment or therapist.

So, an END therapist empowers a client to embody an anti-fragile disposition. This enables a reduced reactivity to the sensations interpreted as fear.[10] In this way, the therapist provides a client with the second perspective of feeling safe,[11] while ensuring that there are limited environmental concerns and so on (i.e. the first perspective of feeling safe). The combination of the two might be considered the essence of therapy itself, at least as far as helping to establish a balanced autonomic nervous system[12] goes.

In the therapeutic setting, these two forms of safety are provided by offering a calm, receptive and quiet environment, and a touch which helps a client to feel whole and able to explore and express health, while being less and less hindered by protective fear, which becomes less and less necessary.

Clients are often surprised at how mere touch can enable such a radical shift in their well-being, and many wonder what it is that we are doing.

Q1: How do we accomplish these effects by offering touch in this way?

Q2: Are we actually 'doing' anything other than touching to provide the feeling of being safe?

An individual's neuroceptivity[13] will greatly appreciate an approach from a therapist that is not agitated, reactive or controlling and will also generally relax within a calm environmental ambience. In other words, their body will feel safe enough to be met with touch. A factor of particular interest, which is somewhat unique to an END therapist's contact, is the ability to provide sensitive openness to whatever presents itself. This non-judgemental and space-enabling openness encourages the gradual dissipation of a client's subconscious reactions to help their system accommodate a wider array of emergent experiences, without being overwhelmed or reacting with defence or avoidance.

In our primitive past, these subconscious reactions were the tendencies sanctioning the body-mind to respond, sustain and optimize the survival of our body in relevant situations. Yet in the manic contemporary world, our physiology gets over-stimulated and as a result the survival responses have become reactive habits often covered and disguised by other reactive habits.

It is the surfacing and revealing of these habits which provide the opportunity for the tendencies underpinning them to be re-evaluated and the potency they have been storing to be freed and re-integrated.

During this process, the therapist's touch is non-verbally saying, 'It's okay to feel these things; actually, it's very helpful to feel them.' With this kind of touch we are encouraging, and indeed empowering, the client not to react to the experience, by non-verbally sharing their sensate experience and creating space for it to be expressed, culminating in stillness being able to reflect the calmness inherent in their being.

In effect we, as END practitioners, reflect calmness by not reacting. Not reacting to what? To the client's tendencies of reacting. By not reacting we are not doing anything to support the reality of any of their surfacing tendencies. We are sensitively sharing our awareness of a client's reactivity, in addition to non-verbally implying that it's okay to be aware of what's unfolding. This 'okaying' helps a client to become familiar, rather than getting fearful, agitated or dissociating from any sensations presenting themselves. Once there is awareness and familiarity with what was previously hidden, in the presence of a trustworthy other, it is no longer subconscious and, therefore, no longer a reaction.

In other words, by acknowledging and establishing non-doing, a therapist enables a client's physiology to re-appraise contact[14] and sensation as something fulfilling and enhancing, rather than something to react to and close off from. This enables subtler patterns of experience to surface from deep within the body matrix.

Biodynamic craniosacral therapists translate this surfacing and balancing as the settling and reintegration of 'potency' and the breath of life within tissues and fluids. This changing nature is the process Dr Sutherland was probably referring to as 'transmutation'.

CLINICAL NOTE

The kind of contact that the therapist offers needs to be preceded by appropriate verbal/non-verbal dialogue. This provides the client with the assurance of safe and relevant expectancy whereby the client has a level of knowing what to expect following on from what is explained by the therapist and/or what is remembered as a felt-sense insight from previous sessions. Having said that it is also important for the provided expectations to be an anchor, but not ball and chain, which goes back to understanding the difference between vault safety and fluid anti-fragile safety.

◆ EXPERIENTIAL EXERCISE 2

Anti-fragile

This is not an exercise to provide to a client, at least not to begin with. It is to help get a handle on the feeling of safety from an anti-fragile perspective.

◆ Start to breathe in and out intentionally through the nostrils (if breathing through the nose is not possible then breathe through the mouth). Keep the eyes relaxed but slightly open.

◆ When reaching the end of the out-breath, immediately breathe back in, and when reaching the end of the in-breath, immediately breathe out again.

◆ Continue with this pauseless cyclic breathing pattern and make it full and slightly audible.

◆ After a minute of breathing in this way, continue but close the eyes and notice if the visual impressions (formed from the visual input the moment before closing the eyes) are still observable in your mind.

◆ Carry on breathing in this fashion, continuous, audible and full, for a few minutes and sustain the awareness of the impressions, if possible. When it is no longer possible, notice how the dissipation of the impressions either gets replaced by other mental impressions, or turns into body sensations (it will be one or the other). If it seems like both occur at the same time then pay closer attention to the quick transition which takes place as the mental impression(s) morph into sensation(s) and vice versa.

◆ Keeping the eyes closed, come back to normal breathing (non-doing breath).

◆ Notice how the impressions of the mind have decreased and the sensations of the body are more present and expressive.

◆ Open the eyes and notice the quality of the perception of vision.

◆ This experiential exercise is an example of doing (breath control) while noticing the subtle non-doing transition which takes place when objectified impressions change to sensations.

◆ After this exercise, the sense of vision often seems as if it is more intimate with the felt-sense of the body and is less agitating to the mind. In other words, we can sense being more in relationship with the environment, while feeling less fragmented and, therefore, less fragile.

Q: Is this all that we are providing – non-reactivity to a client's reactive tendencies?

Actually, no, the bigger part of what we offer is the safe touch enabled by not reacting to *our own* tendencies of reacting. The kind of touch provided from this form of equanimity has a huge effect on a client's system. This is because, unfortunately, it is rare to be touched in this way. Consequentially, this kind of touch helps the client's body feel like it has been met and their ANS often re-balances itself as a result. In other words, by not reinforcing a client's subconscious tendency to sustain/alter or contract/withdraw from an experience, consciousness is provided with a chance to reassimilate itself free from reactive content. Moreover, by being aware and not reacting to our own tendencies (to judge, label, categorize, distract, protect, mobilise, immobilise, etc.), we empower the client to feel safe enough for their system to unfold more deeply and insightfully (see Appendix 2).

Nevertheless, a therapist is susceptible to subconsciously reacting to these tendencies (as they have formed because of a habitual desire to affirm identity) and everything which is bound to them, such as impressions, memory fragmentation, expectations, patterns of experience. The culmination of this desire is 'intention' and a client will, consciously or subconsciously, feel intention in our system, just as we consciously or subconsciously feel it in theirs.[15] So, perhaps the most revelational, indeed transformative, aspect of our therapy occurs when we realize the tendencies in ourselves, and don't react to them. Not only does this awareness and non-reactivity cut off the fuel of intention, it also opens us up to the felt-sense origin of health, due to feeling the changing nature of our sensations and thoughts.[16] That's a game-changing perspective! This perspective will from here on be referred to as 'insight'.

Awareness of and equanimity towards our own tendencies to react, therefore, facilitates both expression and insight of our original nature[17] (original health) by feeling the essence of the ever-changing and vibrant quality of sensation and thought. This insight encourages the dissipation of our intention to change or sustain something, thereby enabling us to witness and resonate with the nature of change itself.[18] The result of witnessing and not reacting to our own sensations and thoughts (i.e. perceiving their changing nature) coaxes the fruition of balance, coherence and the expression of health within a client's system.[19] This culminates in helping the client to feel met, acknowledged and safe, at an essentially subtle level.

Try this: Sit in stillness and let the last paragraph percolate for a bit. The longer we invite stillness in this way the more that the inherent subtle sensations will present themselves, and the feeling of being nurtured by our original nature will become more familiar.

2.2 Familiarity with space and stillness

What you are looking for is what is looking.

ST FRANCIS OF ASSISI

This is the notion that what we are searching for is actually the very essence of who we are. In our practice, the term 'non-doing' is commonly used to describe the undercurrent of this essential aspect of our work. Yet the profound reality of it is rarely understood. To understand it we must first inquire deeply into our own source of presence, referred to here as our original nature.

Again, original nature is a term used to describe our quintessential source, the expression of which we might refer to as 'health'.[20] Health, in this context, does not have an opposite and, therefore, doesn't lend itself to any concept born from duality.[21] If we were to try and conceptually separate original nature from anything else then it would become, at best, an object projected by an individual, deemed to be separate from it. This is a concept based on the impression of duality, not original nature.

Original nature is a 'ground of divisionless movement'; a vibration of emptiness while, paradoxically, being full with the essence of everything. The twentieth-century sage, Jiddu Krishnamurti,[22] attempted to convey its nature as both the source of calm stillness and the essence of intensity. Professor David Bohm, Krishnamurti's student and friend, referred to this dynamic stillness as 'the unlimited', which only has a limit in that it has no limits.[23]

Embodying the paradoxical nature of dynamic stillness causes us to drop the habitual use of identifying language, leaving our original nature and wholistic expression to be felt in its place. If we are in contact with our original nature, the identifiable organismic structure, our body, is still present and locatable, but the insight of dynamic stillness opens a potential beyond the limitations of individual tendencies, impressions, memories and expectations (TI/ME). The awareness of our original nature is, therefore, not the absence of awareness, it is the awareness of TI/ME transitioning to wholeness (i.e. awareness of the passing of psychologic time[24] and the presence of unbounded potential and expression).

Words, which evoke and imply the feeling of separation,[25] cloud the experiential[26] quality of dynamic stillness. It is for this reason that much of this book may at first appear complex in its terms, or perhaps labyrinthine.[27] Try to persevere through these paragraphs, as it will start to become clear that the sentences are just inviting consciousness to stretch itself[28] enough to let go of rutted concepts and to be aware of subtle body-mind sensations. The seeming complexity will dissolve following the insight gleaned from perceiving the changing nature of these sensations. This is what the words are ultimately pointing at – the felt-sense of arising and passing.

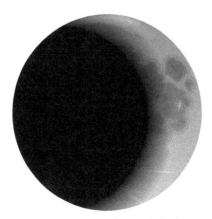

Figure 2.3: The moon of our original nature

Complicated is the pointing finger, simpler than simple is the moon.

If simple words take themselves to be the moon, then it is better to remain complicated.

At least that way a point will be reached where one gives up on thought providing an answer.

The relevance for this approach, in the therapeutic setting, will be discussed in greater detail later in the book. But for now, suffice it to say that when a therapist can release the trajectory of concepts, tendencies, impressions, expectations and so on, then the likelihood of staying stuck in a cyclic loop of intention will diminish. Many body therapists employ multitudes of varying techniques to help change this or that condition in the clients they treat. However, the really deep changes seem to take place once the attempts to change things have ceased, and where health is given the space it needs to express itself.

The following simile may be useful to explain why this is so. Inserting an ignition key in the ignition and turning the key is a well-known method for starting a car engine. It is as if the car remembers how to hum into action once you remind it of its operative nature by turning the key. However, if there is too much fuel in the ignition system, the engine does not start. The more you try to start the car the worse the problem becomes. By simply remaining calm, and waiting for the engine to settle, you will find that the engine will eventually balance whereby the key can be used to start it again.

The settling process in a biologic being is significantly affected by the presence of another biologic being. In the therapeutic setting, a client's engine (physiology) is listening out for subtle references which imply safety while the therapist reminds their system of its own inherent nature (humming). If a therapist intentionally tries to change things it will be like the driver turning the ignition key once the engine is in motion, and will thus cause friction and flooding.

So, the difference with a biologic system, compared to a car, is that after a while there is no need to turn a key for the deep intelligence of the body to remember how to express itself. This is because the body's intelligence mostly needs supporting, instead of being substituted by somebody's intent to evoke change.

Some bodyworkers travel far and wide to learn how to turn the metaphoric ignition key in different ways, developing various techniques and methods. This book may provide some relief for that, first because the majority of the book is about deepening the awareness of your own being as a therapist, and second, because techniques are utilized here as a brief entry point and then relinquished as the potency of the client's system is acknowledged for what it is.

The simile of starting or flooding the car engine may provide enough understanding for the mind to appreciate the relevance of non-doing. However, this simplicity is not it, as it is actually only another concept. While a concept can lend itself to understanding the need for relinquishing habitual tendencies, intentions, expectations and so on, the therapist's mind will likely formulate another technique, albeit disguised, in this case by conceptualizing the vibration of a car engine and imagining it echoing through the body. This is a valid attempt to deepen one's understanding and, who knows, it may eventuate in the insight which has been mentioned, but it is far more likely to result in yet another reactive tendency/intention loop. So this book will outline the reactive tendencies and habits which fuel intention, and will endeavour to investigate this, in a manner deeper than the superficial varnish of conceptual simplicity, by delving into the experiential world of the felt-sense.

Note: Keep referring to the endnotes at the back of this book to aid with the understanding of the terminology and any apparent complexity. Another way of clarifying the paradoxical nature of a phrase such as 'original nature' might be by way of allegory or metaphor. The koan[29] below attempts to illustrate the profundity of our original nature, and how one needs to appreciate the mind's limiting nature before insight of our original nature is revealed. It has been used by teachers in the Chinese Buddhist *ch'an*,[30] Korean *son* and Japanese *zen* traditions for centuries:

Show me your original face.

The face you had before your grandparents were born.

This conundrum appears most famously in case 23 of the koan collection called the 'gateless gate',[31] in which a monk called Myō is extremely jealous that the sixth chan patriarch, Enō, has received the master's robe and bowl. He chases him through the valleys and mountains to take them back, by force if needed. When Myō catches up with Enō he places the robe and bowl on the ground and invites Myō to take them. Yet Myō finds that they are too heavy to lift. Overwhelmed with embarrassment, he asks to be given the teaching instead. Enō responds by saying: 'Without thinking good or bad, in this precise moment, what is your original face? The face you had before your grandparents were born?'

Actually, this koan isn't conceptually that hard. It's like asking a tree what it was before it was a tree, or the wind before it was wind. However, the koan runs deeper than this conceptual understanding; it is asking the student to feel and reveal what is already present. An authentic meditation master never asks to see something that isn't already present!

The face in question is our original nature, a face which is free from the illusion of time, permanence and separation. When the 'mask' obscuring the face is discarded (noticed[32]) it presents itself as a vibrant felt-sense of arising and passing.[33]

END therapists refer to the revealed face as dynamic stillness. Indeed, it can be called any number of names, but in essence it is our original non-dual nature.

Let's expand on the understanding of this revealed face. Rupert Spira articulates this nicely with the following quote:

If someone were to ask us, relatively speaking, to stand up and take a step towards ourself, in which direction would we turn? We cannot take a step towards ourself, because we are already standing at ourself. Nor indeed can we take a step away from ourself, because we take ourself with us wherever we go.

Likewise for awareness, in order to know itself it doesn't have to do anything or go anywhere. It doesn't have to direct its knowing towards itself, because it is already standing at itself. Awareness is too close to itself to know itself in subject-object relationship.[34]

Q: So, how do we become aware of our original nature and establish non-reactivity without doing anything?

Before we can fully appreciate the awareness and non-reactivity needed to realize dynamic stillness, we must first look into the fundamental factor which hinders the awareness of and equanimity towards our own sensations, thoughts and sense of wholeness, namely 'intention'.

◆ EXPERIENTIAL EXERCISE 3

Dissolution of the matrix

◆ Stand in a relaxed position with feet hip width apart and knees soft.

◆ Place the nails of both hands next to each other so that the largest surface area of the nails is touching and the thumb nails are facing the chest.

◆ Start moving one of the hands backwards and forwards so that the nails of each hand rub against one another.

◆ Keep rubbing, gradually increasing the speed, for one minute.

◆ When you stop rubbing, let the arms and hands relax at the sides of the body.

◆ Feel the vibration echo in the fingers, hands, arms, the whole body and the 'bio-nimbus'.[35]

◆ Be interested in the subtlest of the sensations which are presenting themselves. These sensations are not due to the physical stimulation of the nerves. Rather, they are noticeable because the conditioned perspective of the body recedes when awareness is totally present with the felt-sense of arising and passing.

◆ The body is now perceived, if only momentarily, as a screen of awareness letting the dance of arising and passing display itself free from TI/ME.

Chapter 3

Intention

If the only prayer you ever say in your entire
life is Thank you, it will be enough.

MEISTER ECKHART

3.1 Ramifications of intent

Take a moment to observe yourself. Are you moving, conceptualizing, memorizing, remembering, fidgeting, facilitating, procrastinating, manipulating, behaving, not behaving, ruminating, acting…? If so you are 'doing'. Most of us don't even realize that these habits are born, and supported, by the three pillars of 'I', namely identification, impressions and intention. This is because we identify ourselves with the feeling, outcome and content of these reactive habits. Actually, numerous studies demonstrate that we would prefer to be with these habitual tendencies rather than face doing nothing.[1] This includes tendencies which cause pain!

All intention is a movement away from the current 'experiencing' moment and will therefore obfuscate our present felt-sense.[2] However, if you are aware of merely sensing, feeling, perceiving, experiencing and being, then you are embodied in a field of non-doing (free from intention, even intentional attention dissolves in this awareness).

Bearing this in mind, ask the following question:

- Is it possible to invite a field of non-doing?

> Now try it by observing the changing nature of your bodily sensations – any sensations, gross (solidified) or subtle.[3]

At first, this short awareness exercise can seem quite a challenge, because even the act of trying is doing.[4] However, if we persevere with awareness, gently attentive of the changing nature of our arising sensations, the quality of perception alters, from being influenced by past impressions and future projections, to being fed by presence, free from intention.

Presence of this nature doesn't just involve awareness of sensory input[5] and the arising of its corresponding sensation. It includes insight of the sensation 'passing away'. The insight of sensation passing away is radical because it automatically results in the arising of a fresh and less conditioned sensation, freed somewhat from the identification and conditioning of tendencies, impressions, memory and experience (TI/ME).

In other words, the felt-sense awareness of a sensation passing away does not mean that the sensation ceases per se. It means identification to sensations dissipates to allow space for subtler sensations to arise. Awareness of the subtlest sensations provides non-dual insight.

The felt-sense of these subtle sensations arising is, therefore, dependent on the felt-sense of sensations passing away. When we are aware of this the content of thought[6] (TI/ME) becomes less influential and distracting. Such awareness casts a very different perspective on what we generally call sensations, as their arising and passing are not separated by TI/ME. END therapists call the felt-sense of this *potency* – in other words, being aware of the passing phase of any sensation creates the opportunity for the body-mind to refresh and express health and for non-duality to gradually reveal itself.[7]

It is worthwhile, therefore, for an END practitioner to effortlessly inquire into the passing nature of sensations. Insight from such inquiry will help us to realize that non-doing is not the opposite of doing, just as non-duality is not the opposite of duality. Actually, we might discover that the very 'act'[8] (non-doing awareness of sensations passing) is an act free of intention,[9] which a client's system really appreciates.

3.2 Intention prevents insight

We gain clarity to the importance of orientating to our clients in this way, compared to other ways, by investigating the multifarious fields of body and psychotherapy. There is no paucity of literature conveying the need for us to help clients find stillness within themselves in order to feel healthy. Moreover, a deluge of books and courses declare the importance for a practitioner to engender stillness in themselves so as to promote stillness in another. From there they go on to advocate various methods, techniques, intentions and meditations, which, when looked into, are actually all forms of 'doing'.

Please forgive this repetition but it is good to emphasize that the premise of this book proposes that it is this very doing which prevents the awareness of stillness, in the true biodynamic sense of that word. When we explore the nature of stillness with awareness, free from doing, it will become apparent that it has a dynamic quality to it. This quality is one of arising and passing,[10] free from TI/ME – it is potency itself!

Awareness free from intention, therefore, enables insight into the changing non-dual quality of subtle sensations. Put into biodynamic terms, familiarity with non-doing helps us become sensitively aware of potency and the expression of health.

This awareness can be felt as both calm and intense at the same time, which might seem paradoxical to the mind, but is a huge relief for the body (both therapists and clients). When perceived free from interpretation, this felt-sense calm intensity provides insight, but when it is interpreted by thought it becomes a conceptual paradox[11] and becomes vulnerable to the seeming contradictory distortions of duality, i.e. TI/ME.[12]

To fully understand the felt-sense of calm intensity it is better to first explain what it is not. So, we will begin by exploring different types of intention before attempting to deepen our perceptual and conceptual understanding of non-doing.

Intention is the conditioned basis on which an individual is motivationally responsive or reactive to sensory input, including the content of thought.[13] Conditioning of this nature will be regarded either as intention, intent or 'doing'[14] for the rest of this book.

It is, nevertheless, useful to acknowledge that intention is often needed as a means of reminding ourself to be present and attentive to the general courtesies of interaction and to consciously navigate our body. Moreover, in the therapeutic setting, the intention of moving our hand to a region of initial therapeutic relevance helps a client to feel heard and met.

Furthermore, it would be hard to argue against the benefits obtained by upholding the intention to remain awake and to not overtly react to a client's emotional expressions (especially those which we might deem shocking[15]). Yet, wakefulness and non-reactivity are, potentially, much more present without intention.

Intentional attention could, therefore, be viewed as a reminder for not getting side-tracked by subconscious intentions formed by TI/ME. Such intention acts as a balanced platform to establish relevant initial contact, and to provide a grounded presence, encouraging the client to feel safe.

Q: Does intention hold value beyond this?

Many contemporary self-help authors promote the use of positive intention to act as an ignition to help create a proactive outcome in alignment with individual goals. In other words, the intention is focused and acted on, based on a desired outcome. A trajectory of intention is, therefore, promoting the need to achieve a specific result.

Reliance on intention in this way – projecting a desired result and following a set path to achieve it, rather than being open to perceiving and trusting the body's inherent expressions, regardless of whether they seem 'good' or 'bad' – collapses the potential possibility of health fully expressing itself. Considering this, it could be deduced that clinicians who hold intention in their body-mind will not only limit the optimal expression of health,[16] but will also, ineluctably, prevent insight.

Q: Does this mean we should suppress intention apart from the initial intention of setting up, meeting and helping to orientate the client?

Unfortunately, by suppressing intention the nature of it will continue, in another form, beneath the radar of consciousness. The result of this will be that the tension of intention will remain part of the therapeutic interaction, thus limiting the expression of health.[17] It is, therefore, important to be aware of our explicit and implicit intentions rather than suppress them.

Impressions, identification to experience, fluctuating memories and expectations are psychological antecedents to the tendency of sub-consciously reacting with like or dislike.[18] These reactive evaluations result in a subsequent 'charge of desire' set forth to change, sustain or suppress the impression of a perceived object, person, relationship, activity and so on, thus fuelling an amplification of this desire, here called intention (see Appendix 1).[19]

CLINICAL NOTE

While tutoring trainings in the past I have noticed how the last two minutes of a 20-minute hands-on session can be a most profound learning period for both the student treating and the student on the table, especially for newer students. Health often starts to express itself in a much more evident way during this period. The reason for this is that the student treating is asked by the tutor to find the most appropriate way to end the session over the last couple of minutes. During that window, the stealth intentions often dissipate as the student lets go of the uncon-scious desire to affect the condition of the student on the table. In other words, the student lets go of their subconscious 'doing' (intention).

◆ EXPERIENTIAL EXERCISE 4

Attention to insight
Trataka to *vidya*

- ◆ Use the paper with the black dot.

- ◆ Place it on your lap or at arms length on the table.

- ◆ Look at the black dot without blinking for two minutes.

- ◆ Then close your eyes.

- ◆ What do you notice in your third-eye region?

- ◆ Keep looking at whatever is in that space.

- ◆ Is there any like or dislike with what arises here?

- ◆ Try not to answer this too quickly. It is an opportunity for the mind's tendencies to reveal themselves and for you to notice their passing nature.

- ◆ As space replaces the mind impression, notice the dissolution of the content.

- ◆ Let the dissolution of the impression open you up to the dissolution (laya) of the body sensations. They are ultimately the same!

3.3 Types of intent

There is a gamut of different types of intention which could be described. Moreover, the complexity of the human mind ensures that we
continue to discover more. Nevertheless, in the context of touch-based
therapy, intent can be broken down into six main types of intention,
two forms of intentional attention and one universal intention, which
is 'accessed' via intentional intention:

1. Held intention

2. Directing intention

3. Beguiled intention

4. Grey-zone intention

5. Facilitatory intention

6. Guidance/reassurance-based intention

7. Ground intention.

Two replacements for intention, by awareness 'stretching' itself:

1. Access attention (intentional attention)

2. Invitation.

Held intention

An example of held intent is when tension is held in the hands after
being used repeatedly in actions such as lifting, manipulating or facilitating objects (e.g. using spanners to undo bolts). If we clench our
fist an effort is required, but after some time of holding our hand in
that state the clenched fist will seem to be the natural condition of our
hand and we will no longer be aware of the effort required to maintain
it. If we were to now open our hand it would initially seem that we
needed to make an effort to do so. Such tension, therefore, results
from subconscious intention and becomes stored as a body-based habit
following the sustained input of wilful intention.

CLINICAL NOTE

It is not just our hands that fall prey to the habit of held intent. The whole body can echo with this subconscious tension and, as a result, it becomes a part of the way we structure belief and function in the world.

A very helpful way to simultaneously realize and soften this intent is to practise visualizing a clenched fist and imagine the gradual relaxation of it for approximately one minute. Repeat this a few times. Once you have become familiar with the process then visualize the whole body as clenched and let it release over the same duration, then repeat it as before.

With this type of visualization there is often a realization and release of held intention which provides a wider perceptual field – a perceptual field which was already 'there', only clouded by the habituated tension of covert doing. Feel the space left by the passing away of the tension. In other words, sense the nature of intention dissolving. This opens a whole new way of perceiving the body, which is much more fulfilling.

Clients will react to held intention by reciprocal reaction, i.e. subconscious tension/protection.

A therapist non-doing, in the manner outlined, reduces a client's reactivity, thus their body gets the chance to express health.

Directing intention

Subconsciously held intention often stems from a consciously directed intention. For example, mechanical interventions are incorporated into bodywork therapies due to our understanding of machinery (working parts of something) with which we provide a force to affect the position of the parts. However, a presumption is made when we translate the mechanistic impressions and understanding into the world of body therapy. This is because the understanding formed by mechanical impressions tells us we are merely machines and are nothing but inert matter subject to the mechanical effects conducted by applied force.[20]

Thought, especially western thought, has continued to reinforce the mechanical mindset and, as a result, our rationale for how body-based therapies work is mostly dependent on it.[21] Consequentially, the therapist is conditioned to implement directional force to alter that which is perceived as needing to change. This perspective then seeps into our motivation (motor-based intention) to direct a client's body. Unfortunately, this will engender a 'doing' tension in the therapist's system, and despite this therapy asking a therapist to not 'do' anything,[22] the directing habit is hard to come out of.

To illustrate, a massage therapist who intentionally contracts and relaxes the muscles in their hands, in order to mould and shape various tissues of the client's body, repeats similar movements many times. In so doing, the wilful intention will likely become instinctively reactive and/or automated, to preserve the energy expenditure of the therapist having to consciously think about each individual movement.

From an evolutionary perspective, this kind of intention is likely to have an adaptational advantage in certain environments, due to the repetitious intention becoming less conscious and thus requiring less cerebral energy to maintain the intention. For example, a monkey subconsciously gripping their hand or foot in order to hang from a tree branch for extended periods of time would free up more conscious attention to notice environmental opportunities such as potential food or danger.

However, just because much of a therapist's intention is subconscious, this does not mean that intention has any less impact on the tissues of the client. Such subconscious intention fragments perception due to its nature of maintaining motor output and overriding sensory input. This results in decreased skin and subcutaneous awareness. Furthermore, intention of this kind has a desensitizing effect on the wholistic felt-sense of the therapist and promotes habituated reactivity to stimulus, rather than relational sensitivity.

It is pertinent, therefore, that we become conscious of our own subconscious intentions prior to and during a treatment session (along with equanimity and insight[23]).

In END training sessions, we are reminded again and again that the body knows what to do when the appropriate relational contact is made. Nevertheless, intention held in the therapist's body, due to the repeated use of directed intervention, is often so deeply ingrained that it can take a great many practice sessions and self-awareness exercises before the habit of mechanical intention dissipates fully. Still, with perseverance and patience it does happen.

Beguiled intention

An example of beguiling intent is when one's mind scans either the body of oneself, the client or both, in order to discover and isolate rhythms. Over time, this intent becomes a habit and sets up a trajectory of 'blind intent' and a consequential form of imagination. With this kind of intent, the impression of a rhythm or flow can emerge. Yet, this movement is nothing other than the formulated reflection of the movement of the therapist's own mind. In other words, it is the habituated translation of subtle sensations via the mind's tendency to project an adopted rhythm.[24] Yet, the impression of natural unfacilitated movement may seem very real – as real as the clothes on the metaphoric naked emperor![25]

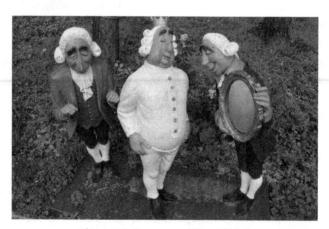

Figure 3.1: Emperor with no clothes

This presents a problem for the therapist, in as far as the intention has not only developed beyond the purpose of a biodynamic platform, but is born from the charge of desire formed by one's own reactive tendencies. Such desire will, by nature, extinguish open curiosity and therefore prevent the insight of change[26] and so cannot be used as a platform for inquiry.[27]

Grey-zone intention

It becomes more problematic when a therapist translates mechanical concepts into 'energetic' intent ('grey-zone' intention). Directing and channelling energy is a very difficult intention to let go of. This is because such intent is both subtle and beguilingly attractive, especially for people who already realize the limitations of mechanical intent but unknowingly wish to remain in control. This grey-area intention can, therefore, have the feeling, to some extent, of a witch or wizard 'healing' the client.

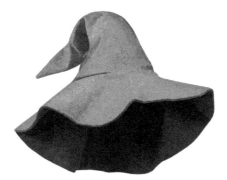

Figure 3.2: Wizard's hat

Not only is this a really tricky intentional base to let go of, but it can also be hard to ascertain the reason *why* one should let go of it at all! This is because the lead up to this kind of intention involves the presence of a certain amount of potency-based awareness, which is useful for encouraging the expression of health. But equanimity, understanding and insight are not present, which means true relational touch is not present and an optimal expression of health is, thereby, not possible.

Awareness and equanimity of potency are like two wings enabling the bird to fly (metaphor for insight). If one wing is operational but the other isn't then the bird will never ascend to the air. The moment one perceives arising and passing as the essential reality of potency then TI/ME and intention cease to exist. If this is not realized then the translation of potency will remain a perspective of duality (observer separate from the observed). This is obviously a hindrance to the felt-sense understanding of non-duality and will consequently inhibit the 'knowing' of dynamic stillness.

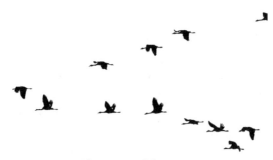

Figure 3.3: Flying cranes

Without a felt-sense understanding of non-duality any equanimity will be transient and, therefore, stop short of providing beneficial insight pertaining to change and the expression of health.

It is very common for therapists who have developed a subtle(ish) awareness of potency to become 'involved' with it. This is ill-fated as such involvement is based on perpetuating intention and will, inevitably, prevent the expression of health from presenting itself fully. This is a grey area as it is obvious that there is only one 'wing' in operation.

Fortunately, therapists trained in the field of END often come to realize this and release the intent held around projecting and wilfully being mesmerized by subtler expressions, such as pseudo-tides and pseudo-midlines.[28] This approach of realizing the habit of inherent intention and releasing it[29] powerfully affects our awareness and equanimity and deeply acknowledges the inherent intelligence within the body.

Q1: Can we, as END practitioners, really be non-intentional when we are aware of this subtlety (fluids, potency, tides, midlines)?

Q2: Or, do we overlay concepts onto the expressions and delude ourselves into believing we are non-doing?

The tides are a potential grey zone for END practitioners as they can be an alluring sign indicating that a client's system is reorganizing and our own awareness is deepening in the process. However, it is portentous not to be transfixed by this expression of health, which requires a fair amount of equanimity. This is because if a tide is not felt for what it is then the mind of the therapist will become enchanted by the tide's 'current', and, while being pleasant and helpful for relaxing into a relational space (so potency can gather), it can also be the source of preventing deeper equanimity. If equanimity does not keep up with awareness then non-dual insight will not present itself. This is a problem well known by many established meditation traditions.[30]

Let's recap here: awareness of sensations passing, equanimity, 'equipresent' perceptual fields and non-dual insight are all needed to be truly non-doing. If they are not all present we are most likely treating with an aspect of intention and are therefore...doing!

The following *ch'an* allegory might help illustrate the situation we face in this grey zone:

Two monks were arguing about a flag.
    One said: 'The flag is moving.'
    The other said: 'The wind is moving.'

Figure 3.4: Flag and pole in wind

The abbot happened to be passing by and overheard them.
    He told them: 'Not the wind, not the flag; mind[31] is moving.'

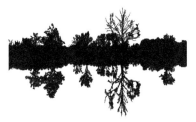

Figure 3.5: The still mind sees clearly

Commentaries on this story note that the mind (TI/ME) is in and of itself a movement based on intention, whereas 'no mind'[32] is the paradox of both movement and stillness free of intention and, therefore, operating from non-doing.

The most difficult expressions for us to develop equanimity towards are the subtle pleasant ones. Not reacting to the gross unpleasant sensations, such as pressure, tightness, tension, pain and heaviness, is a piece of cake compared to not reacting to pleasant sensations.[33] Check it out.

We are socially conditioned to want more of what is perceived as pleasant. This includes the expressions which appear as tides of fluidity and potency. When aware of subtlety, the doing habits of the mind want to get involved with the felt-sense of arising and passing and do something with it. If the mind were not to get involved then the essence of subtle expressions, such as the 'tides', would provide awareness of sensation passing more than arising (P>A; see Appendix 1), and therefore help open to the felt-sense non-doing interface between the relative and the absolute. The felt-sense understanding of the last sentence is insight.

This is not dynamic stillness, it is the calm yet intense 'state' which reflects dynamic stillness (the ground[34]), that which is non-dual. It is an interface between dynamic stillness and the primary midline of physiologic organization and sensory differentiation.

Appreciating this, as body-based therapists, it might be dawning on us that, despite treating efficiently in the way we have been taught, we might not be enabling the full depth and potential of what our particular therapy has to offer. And the reason for this is due to our overriding intentions which react with doing and prevent non-doing.

Another issue presents itself within this metaphoric grey zone and that is the issue of 'preference'. If the therapist surreptitiously starts preferring a particular state over what the client's system is wishing to express, then the therapist's subtle inclination to like and dislike will further prevent equanimity and, therefore, limit the insight of non-duality and non-doing.

This is because when a thought based on an object is liked or disliked the feeling and memory become one and stored in the body as a potential sensation and in the mind as an impression.[35] It now resides as a merry-go-round of reactive tendencies and goes towards forming and sustaining what we (END therapists) call patterns of experience.

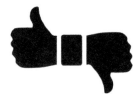

Figure 3.6: Like and dislike

When one is aware of this pattern, and settles into it, it can be perceived as sensations which we either desire more or less of. However, if there is enough awareness of the tendency, and if the reactive pattern is given space to reintegrate into the natural expressions as a whole, this will enable the perception of the sensations to neither be liked or disliked. Many cultures and traditions provide words for such subtle neutral sensations. Yet, the very naming of this expression will separate it from the experiencer and therefore promote a dualistic perception (followed by the associated reactive tendencies). Nevertheless, we call 'it' potency to placate the mind's yearning for a noun and let it dissolve into a verb as realization increases.

Facilitatory intention

The use of gentle guidance by a therapist's hands has been a key principle incorporated by the predecessors of craniosacral therapy practice, especially since Dr William Sutherland first introduced cranial osteopathy. The therapist listens (non-intentionally feels) to the body with openness and interest while incorporating manual facilitation to the bones, joints and adjoining tissues, thus encouraging rhythmic movement to structures which may have become restricted.

This was a unique contribution to the world of body therapy as it was perhaps the most notable time (at least in the west) that listening to the body was prioritized over doing something in order to change the body. Nonetheless, there is still intention to change something in the client's body. This intention follows very soon after the therapeutic listening, often by exaggerating the vector of ease and/or 'inducing' a still point in the client's body. This approach became more popular and well known when Dr John Upledger verified its efficacy and added to the technical component of various hand holds and directions for applying intent.

The technical precision and intention to facilitate a mechanical movement are distinctive features which are relinquished in biodynamic practice, as it becomes clear that reintegration of experiential patterns are due to the body's inherent intelligence, not intervention.

Many therapists, utilizing facilitatory intention, argue that some clients need to feel that something is being 'done' in order to relax and feel confident in the presence of the practitioner. However, a counter argument offered, usually by biodynamic craniosacral practitioners, is that the only reason for a client needing an intervention-based excuse in order to feel something is because the client feels a lack of connection and safety.

So this kind of intentionality could be a help or a hindrance for the client. If it is helpful for the client then it can certainly be helpful for us as the therapist to reduce our own default patterns of intention. For example, we can start to facilitate the slowing down of the breath by intentional nose breathing and slightly contracting the muscles of the naso-oral pharynx during the out-breath. After a while practising this we might realize that we don't need to continue with this intention, as the breath will naturally balance to the needs of the environment and physiologic demand when body awareness is established. Therefore, the initial intention is really only to help the mind settle and to help the body to be aware of its needs.

Try the subtle fasting of the breath exercise in Chapter 7 (Access Attention) to help experientially understand this.

Guidance/reassurance-based intention

This kind of intention is the goal-oriented focus used by many exercise-prescribing therapists such as physiotherapists and yoga therapists. It is the tactile guidance and reassurance used to complement the therapist's vocal instruction, helping a client to adopt various postures, exercises and breathing techniques (etc.) (see Chapter 12, Cranioga). The therapist's hands are used mostly to help a client isolate a particular area of their body and to provide the comfort of tactile contact. An aspect of directing and facilitatory intention is often amalgamated into this intention, which can itself be reassuring for the new client. However, this also means that the therapist must have a way of accessing their own awareness of TI/ME passing. This is because an aspect of both directing and facilitatory intention will, at some point, transition from being conscious to being subconscious, and thus drag the therapist into 'blind TI/ME'. Access attention acts as an antidote to this happening, and this will be explained towards the end of this chapter.

◆ HANDS-ON EXERCISE 1

Noticing intention and letting it go

◆ Working in pairs, start with the hands at the feet.

◆ Notice the feeling of the client's body that unfolds with this intention.

◆ Now come to the awareness of the touch of the breath as it passes through your nostrils for one minute (still in contact with the client's feet).

◆ Then come to the awareness of tongue touch for a minute.

◆ Come into the awareness of tympanic touch (only sound) for a minute.

◆ Now retinal touch (only sight) for a minute.

◆ Finally, come to the awareness of skin touch (only touch, whole-body touch) for one minute and after a minute come back to the awareness of the client with the awareness of the touch of your whole body.

◆ With this contact do you notice the irrelevance of intent?

◆ Recall the initial contact when you applied intention.

◆ How does the client system feel different?

3.4 Ground intention, access attention and invitation
Ground intention

Until now we have explored intention formed by the desire born from a reactive mind. Now we'll mention intent born from nature beyond the mind, which can sound pseudo-scientific or perhaps even poetic at times, especially to ardent materialists. This is because the way we generally perceive intention is to identify its source as either deriving from me, her, him, them or it, and so on. However, nature's intent cannot be isolated in this manner. Actually, the only way to identify its source is to surrender to the fact that we cannot isolate it and appreciate it as a ground of dynamic stillness which manifests as form. So, the 'ground' intent is to manifest itself. Biodynamic craniosacral therapists refer to this process of manifestation as the breath of life and it is from the ground of potential that health and body intelligence express themselves.

If we conceptualize stillness as being separate from the potentially mobile nature of form, it appears as if stillness is opposite to motion. However, insight reveals that stillness, in this context, is in fact also dynamic, but not in the way that thought dualistically perceives stillness and motion. So, the intent of the groundswell of potential is not the mobilizing intention brought about by thought, rather it is presenting its true nature in a way that reveals a dynamically still quality. Realizing and embodying this is the insight of engaged non-doing.

Non-doing sounds easy for us to 'incorporate' into a treatment session, and it is not uncommon for many practitioners to think we just need to be still and quieten our minds and, *voila*, we are non-doing. Yet, the reality of what is meant by non-doing requires a calm and dedicated inquiry into the felt-sense of intention (doing) before there can be an appreciation of what non-doing really implies. Following with this perspective it may, at some point, be realized that the engaged felt-sense inquiry into doing...*is* non-doing! Put another way, engaged non-doing (END) reveals intention for what it is. Awareness of, and equanimity towards, the sensations primed by intention eventually unveils a felt-sense paradox of calm intensity to replace the impression of a solid body, which then reveals 'its' essential nature beyond the impression of a separate body – dynamic stillness. This revelation acts not only as a gateway to realizing 'ground intent' but also to perceiving the changing nature of nature – i.e. what is sometimes referred to as potency, chi, prana and so on.

Access attention[36]

Access attention (intent-derived attention), in the context of END therapy, is conscious orientation to an area of the body brought about by the initial desire to achieve the specific result of relinquishing the binding nature of intention (conscious and subconscious), thereby providing enough space, safety and stillness for the body to feel able to express itself. In this way, the 'noble desire', forming attention, is, in essence, focused awareness (*attendere*[37]) on a specific area of the body, to help sensations show themselves (Specific Area of Sensation Awareness, SASA[38]).

This helps awareness to sense the passing of TI/ME,[39] providing an opportunity to reveal and relinquish intention, including the initial noble desire incorporated by the applied attention.

In END practice, we are aware that conscious mechanically directed intention, used to apply a treatment intervention, is too solid for the sensitivity needed to perceive the health-promoting subtle expressions of the body. So we gently discard this approach, as and when it is appropriate; in other words, when relevant guidance-based intention is no longer necessary. As mentioned, this does not mean that we relinquish intention entirely, at least not as an initial part of the treatment, when it can act as a platform to help the clients' appreciation for non-doing and enhance our own awareness.

For example, the initial intention used to set up the environment to optimize the provision of safe touch is a hugely helpful form of intention, although it is not needed once a safe relational field is established. Another example is the intention of listening to a client speak. The listening often starts as a motor act by contracting certain intrinsic ear muscles. The act of listening, therefore, begins as a motor intention (a form of facilitatory intention). When an interesting conversation progresses, the attention becomes effortless and engaged non-doing replaces the motor intention – the motor is humming without the need to keep turning the ignition key.

So, the access attention (initial intention and sustained attention) promotes orientation, which can open to insight, which then relinquishes the need for intention.

An example of access attention, which can be very useful, is that of attuning our felt-sense to the philtrum of our upper lip and letting the natural non-doing touch of the breath unveil the sensations of our skin in that region. This can encourage the whole body to show itself and consequentially develop a relational field necessary for the client's system to show itself. This particular example will be expanded on later, as it is a generically useful spot for accessing the initial insight of subtle sensations arising and passing.[40]

These access areas act as a platform for attentively letting go of the initial intention and help the therapist to become aware of the subtle felt-sense needed for the insight of TI/ME passing. Intentions beyond this are inevitably fuelled, and reacted upon, by a synthesis of knowledge, tendencies, impressions and memories which one has accumulated from past experiences and projected to form expectations. In other words, the make-up of what is deemed to be 'me', deciding what should or should not be changed, is an amalgamation of knowledge in a maze of reactive habits, the two being inseparable from one another. So, 'my' intention will always involve some form of projection based upon a desire fed by something other than the relational felt-sense of the present situation.

Intent-derived attention, therefore, is different from reactively fuelled intention, in that it can be used to gain access and orientate to the body's intelligence. Listening to the body's intelligence is the real key to acknowledging and adapting to the individual's needs and helping their potential for their patterns of experience to surface and express themselves. This is 'done' while the therapist does nothing apart from remaining aware, not needing to achieve a particular result. Moreover, minimal 'talk therapy' is needed, as the body intelligence is calling the shots. Any form of wilful intention (including talk therapy) will overshadow the intelligence of the body if not relinquished soon after biodynamic expressions are felt. So, perceiving and acknowledging the ephemeral nature of intention is of key importance.[41]

Invitation

Once access attention has opened to the sense, and understanding, of bodily sensations arising and passing, the therapist is in a position to invite various perceptual fields on a spectrum from narrow to wide. The benefit of having established this awareness and understanding is that there is no need to fixate on a particular field.

In this situation, intention turns to attention and open inquiry. Interestingly, the therapist who promotes a relational field such as this is often in touch with what the body might need and is in a position to non-verbally ask the body what it needs and whether it requires narrow or wide fields to join the 'party'.[42] This is, in effect, open felt-sense invitation, not intention. Invitation of this nature can help encourage a client's system to open into more subtlety.

For example, the therapist might invite the bones of the skull to soften in order for the fluid expression of the body to unfold. Invitation of this kind can also be used to help the client's system to calm down, or wake up. It is important to note here that this is not intention, as the therapist is neutral to there being a particular outcome. However, it is also useful to be cautious to the fact that any invitation involving expectation is an intention in disguise. Suspecting the potential for change is not expectation, it is an experienced practitioner knowing to surrender to possibilities while recognizing felt-sense themes.

◆ EXPERIENTIAL EXERCISE 5

Gazing and breath attention
Options
NOSE TIP GAZE (*NASIKAGRA DRISHTI*)

◆ Sitting comfortably, direct your eyesight to the nose tip.

◆ It will feel as though you are going cross-eyed.

◆ One side of the nose will be noticed more than the other.

◆ See if you can balance the awareness by looking through the eye which has less nose tip in its vision.

◆ Spend half a minute here, then spend ten seconds with the other eye.

◆ Keep swapping the eyes with this ratio of visual duration.

◆ After a few minutes, see if the nose tip can be seen with both eyes.

◆ This is a useful exercise for eyesight balancing and ocular muscle release. It is good for easing agitation in a hyped-up system (good for rajasic temperaments).

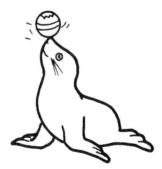

Figure 3.7: Nose tip attention

THIRD-EYE GESTURE (*SHAMBHAVI MUDRA*)

◆ Direct your vision towards the space between the eyebrows.

◆ You will just notice the curved silhouette of the orbital aspect of the frontal bone.

◆ One curve will be more prominent than the other.

◆ See if you can balance the awareness by looking through the eye which has less orbit curve in its vision.

◆ Spend half a minute here, then spend ten seconds with the other eye.

◆ Keep swapping the eyes with this ratio of visual duration.

◆ After a few minutes, see if the curves can be seen with both eyes.

◆ This is a useful exercise for eyesight balancing and ocular muscle release. It is good for invigorating a system which is lacking spark (good for tamasic temperaments).

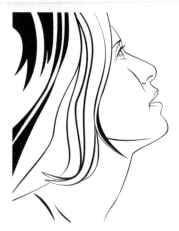

Figure 3.8: Third-eye attention

TOUCH OF BREATH AWARENESS (*ANAPANA*)

◆ Breathe through the nose if possible.

◆ Notice the natural breath leaving the nostrils with exhalation.

◆ Notice the natural breath entering the nostrils with inhalation.

◆ Which nostril is the breath passing? Left or right or both nostrils together?

◆ Is the natural breath shallow or deep?

◆ Is there a sense of temperature difference on the inside of the nostrils when you breathe in compared to when you breathe out?

◆ Do you get a sense of the touch of the breath on the inside of the nostrils?

◆ Do you get a sense of the touch of the breath on the philtrum of the upper lip above cupid's bow?[43]

◆ If you do notice the touch of the breath on the philtrum of the upper lip, how long can you be aware of this without being distracted by thoughts, feelings or emotions?

◆ If you are aware here for longer than one minute without being distracted, do you notice any subtle sensation?

◆ If you can sense a subtle sensation here, is there insight of the sensation arising and passing?

◆ This is a useful exercise for opening up the subtle sensation awareness of the whole of the body and good for accessing a state of balanced awareness (often accessed easiest by those with more sattvic temperaments).

Figure 3.9: Philtrum attention

TI/ME Passing

*And while I stood there I saw more than I can tell and
understood more than I saw; for I was seeing in a sacred
manner the shapes of all things in the spirit, and the shape
of all shapes as they must live together like one thing.*

BLACK ELK

4.1 TI/ME

TI/ME[1] is an acronym which stands for tendencies,[2] impressions,[3] memories[4] and expectations[5] and highlights the formation of the relative self (I/Me). These are the major ingredients culminating to form conditioned thoughts and thinking, as well as becoming a by-product of thought. Yet, TI/ME[6] is *not* the essence of thought per se. TI/ME is the essence of conditioning which generally feeds thought and vice versa. The 'content of thought', which is TI/ME, fuels the intention to evaluate, organize and identify with 'things'.

To elaborate, the content of thought always separates what is perceived based on the past, then it modifies it in the 'present', and then projects it into the future. In other words, thought can never describe 'now' without it being a modification of the past.

Knowing this helps us realize what the past really is. It is an accumulation of reactive tendencies, impressions, identification, interpretations, intentions, implicit and explicit memories, expectations and body-based experiences, i.e. TI/ME with an emphasis on the 'I' – get the gist of the cycle?

TI/ME and body sensations cannot be separated, actually they are the same. It is thought fuelled by TI/ME which gives the impression of division and separates the body from the mind.

It is actually TI/ME which prevents the expression of the subtlest sensations (potency).[7] In addition to this, TI/ME continues the habit-based motion of the mind,[8] no matter how subtle the mind's rhythm may appear.[9]

It should be clarified here that TI/ME is, of course, vital for our ability to associate and practically orientate as an individual being in the world. This individual sense could be considered the limit which the unlimited was missing.

As we are developing beings, endowed with an adapting nervous system, TI/ME helps us co-regulate with primary caregivers. It helps to build appropriate attachments to people and objects which enable us to safely encounter and engage with society. TI/ME, therefore, encourages and establishes developmental attachment processes from the womb through to adulthood. When this does not occur, an individual's system can become disordered. However, when an individual's nervous system has developed in a secure manner, feeling safe to engage with society, TI/ME continues to get used[10] as a tool to sustain our adaptability with the world.

So, we explore the world with the tool and fuel of TI/ME. Yet it is this very tool which cyclically stymies our ability to 'enter' the subtle depths of felt-sense connection, despite our utilizing it to practically orientate and protect ourselves as an organism. What a dilemma!

Q: What can we do to become aware of the habit of TI/ME?

Thought objects (identified impressions) are considered a distraction from insight awareness during a treatment session and so we generally ignore them. However, as mentioned, the reactive tendencies associated with these impressions continue to prevent the felt-sense insight of arising and passing and therefore limit the expression of potency.

We cannot extract a thought or feeling, the same way that we cannot pluck a dream from the mind. Nevertheless, we can become aware of the inherent nature of thoughts and feelings – the sensations they exhibit (due to intention) and the felt-sense which is perceived when they pass away. Such noticing presents sensations as the substrate of impressions and provides insight into their passing nature. Insight of this kind, therefore, emancipates awareness both from identifying with impressions and from the cyclical intentions which sustain TI/ME. It also opens awareness to TI/ME's original nature, non-duality.[11] See Appendix 1 for an expansion on this.

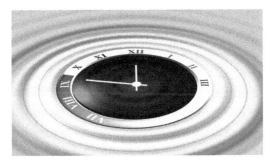

Figure 4.1: Time dissolving into wholeness

4.2 Noticing

Look at the flow chart in Appendix 1. The place where passing of TI/ME is initially, and most effectively, noticed is at the level of body sensations, as will now be explained.

Sensory input

Light, sound, odour, environmental and internal pressure, temperature, neurone activity and so on formulate and fragment consciousness to provide us with an impression of being an individual being conscious.

Impressions (arising[12])

An impression of being an individual being 'conscious' results in validating a 'me'-based experience and having a mind separate from other minds.[13] The knock-on effect from this is that the mind will immediately interpret any sensory input by identifying the source of the input as a cause, i.e. a 'thing'. This objectified experience then promotes a tendency to evaluate, mostly by categorizing it as a liked or disliked experience, which results in a corresponding thought-based reaction.

Noticing the reality of sensory input, without reaction, is an exquisitely subtle 'act' and requires a significant amount of calm presence, which is paradoxically very intense.[14] It is important to note that if the impression causes sufficient dislike then the reactive tendency of an individual will often be to dissociate from the object, whereas if there is sufficient liking towards the object then the tendency will more likely be one of sustaining, repeating, or getting more of the impression. At an even subtler level, the witnessing of these impressions will reveal that the perceived object is associated to the body via the perception of space, and to the mind via the perception of time. Both space and time will seem limited when the prevailing impression is of me being an observer being separate from the observed. However, when there is the perception of impressions passing away, space reveals itself as infinite and time as eternal. In other words, there is only space and there is no time! Although this quality of eternal space cannot be put into words, it is not the same quality of space which we conceive with our minds or dissociate into.

Sensations (Arising and Passing (A+P))

By identifying the source of the sensory input as a separate object, a sensation arises within the body. This provides support for the impressions which are related to body and mind and engenders a loop of continuity (see Appendix 1). In biodynamic craniosacral therapy this is known as a pattern of experience, in Sanskrit it is known as *samskara* (in Pali: *sankhara*).

Yet, it is here that the cycle of TI/ME can provide the deepest insight of passing[15] (P=A) of both body and mind. Nevertheless, if the quality of passing is not realized here, then the impression of the object being separate and permanent will reinforce our sense of duality. This separation will then feed what we generally consider to be consciousness[16] – the 'I'-based perception of the universe. Therefore, it may prove helpful to relinquish naming and labelling sensations, at least after a while. Otherwise the sensations perceived will not provide the insight of TI/ME passing. This is because it is TI/ME which does the naming.

Tendencies (A>P)

Any sensation which lacks the insight of passing promotes the reactive tendency of craving and aversion (including fear) towards the sensation, rather than realizing the essential reality of the sensation. In other words, wanting more, or less, of the sensation is a reactive tendency which will prevent the awareness of TI/ME passing (insight). In the Sanskrit language, this reactive tendency is a point of conditioning known as *vasana*.

The *vasana* is a subtle blend of impressions, evaluations, sensations and intentions. If craving or aversion has arisen in the mind there will be no awareness of the sensation *passing*. This is because the tendency to react with intention has reached the point of no return and will turn into action (skt: *karma*; pli: *kamma*). Tendencies include the orientation, formulation and association of thoughts based on an original experience, and usually result in an individual's perception being funnelled into a limited field of awareness, including states of dissociation.

Intention

The forming intention is the manifestation of an act to either associate and increase a feeling or object, or dissociate from and reduce a feeling or object. However, the precursory tendency of reacting to sensations is not known by the perceiver. This is because the changing nature of the sensation is not being understood and, as a result, potency is inhibited from expressing its inherent quality of arising and passing. Any intention will further enhance and affirm the impression of the sensory input as being a separate object. Therefore the body sensations, arising from the impression, will seem to be perpetually arising and, as a result, interpreted as permanent. Such solid, and seemingly permanent, sensations are often labelled and identified with, by the person perceiving them. They include pain, pressure, heaviness, tightness, tension and so on.

Inhibition of such quality, therefore, forms a charge of desire wanting to change or sustain the impression (object), rather than realize the insight of perceiving change itself. The felt-sense of change (skt: *tanmatra*) free from TI/ME provides the insight of arising being the same as passing (A=P) – non-dual.[17] This is real felt-sense non-duality rather than the conceptual or dissociated form of 'non-duality'.

This all might seem complex – and that is because the content of thought *is* very complex, whether it is as a result of reading this or not. At least when one yields to the unfathomable nature of this subject then thought realizes its own inherent limits. That way, one notices that, beyond these limits, the essence of thought and sensations is akin to the dynamic dance of light intimate with the still TV screen. This subject then reveals itself as very, very simple – so simple in fact that when insight dawns we realize that we were missing it because of trying to understand it!

◆ EXPERIENTIAL EXERCISE 6

Passing
Abbaya

◆ Notice the different temperature inside your nostrils when you breathe in compared to when you breathe out.

◆ Be present and aware of the sensations inside the nostrils that are more subtle than the sense of temperature.

◆ Let your awareness acknowledge the rest of the body at this level of subtlety.

◆ In this way, the sensations can be felt with more appreciation of their inherent nature of both arising and passing. With this perceptive awareness, the conditioned nature of TI/ME starts to dissolve.

◆ The longer you persevere with this awareness, despite any uprising of grosser sensations, the more the passing quality will be emphasized and there will be less emphasis on the quality of arising – until a point is reached where there is a balance between arising and passing, free of TI/ME.

CLINICAL NOTE

At such point a stilling will pervade through the body-mind. This is a still point.

A still point is where there is a re-sourcing of the client's system concurrent with the therapist accessing insight (see Chapter 6, Calm In-10-City).

This insight and understanding enable dynamic stillness to be a felt-sense realization rather than a nebulous conceptual paradox based on a distorted impression of consciousness.

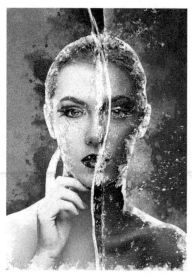

Figure 4.2: Subtle body: waking to the passing of TI/ME

4.3 Change

Perceptual fields, tides, tissue, fluid and a midline expression are felt-sense revelations which enable an END practitioner to encourage health in a grounded and safe manner. But, within all of this, it is perceiving and understanding potency which provides the insight of change.[18]

Potency is often spoken in the same vein as *prana, chi, ki* or *rlung,* stemming from understanding and practices in various countries (especially those in Asia). However, potency may be a word which is set up better for impartial inquiry, especially for more western understanding. This is because the word potency is less established as a noun than the other words, and thus promotes itself as more of a verb. Actually, the word *dhamma* (skt: *dharma*) is even better, as the investigation underpinning this word goes so deep into the source of nature that, when fully understood, the observer, act of observation and the observed are perceived as no longer separate. Nevertheless, the word potency has been used more than the word *dhamma* in the contemporary bodywork literature, so we will run with that word for now.

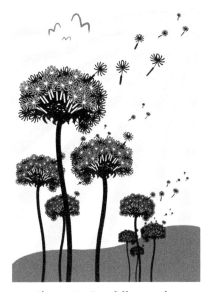

Figure 4.3: Dandelion passing

Q: Why mention this?

Because any mind-based objectification of what potency implies will obscure non-dual insight, as will now be explained.

What if we could slow down the felt-sense of potency? If we could we would notice it comprises of two essential qualities: 1) arising and 2) passing. To better describe potency, as a sensation, let us replace the word potency with the word 'tingling'.[19] With only two syllables, instead of three, tingling can be used to illustrate the arising and passing qualities of potency. The 'tin' syllable represents the arising, and the 'gling' syllable represents the passing.

Placing the emphasis on the gling will help the arising (tin) to be freed from the impression it is conditioned by. Persevering with gling, as if it were a mantra, has potential to engender a still point. This enables a greater sense of wholeness and a sense of fresh arising (tin). Eventually the arising and the passing will be no different, which will provide insight as the non-dual 'tone' of consciousness.

The felt-sense passing vibration of potency can be especially noticed in the body at the umbilical/small intestine, heart and third ventricle regions due to these regions being functionally used for subtle transformation, such as food to nutrients, centre of gravity to balance, impulse to beat, blood to CSF.

◆ EXPERIENTIAL EXERCISE 7

Sound passing
Mantra japa

- ◆ Bring to mind the word 'tingling'.

- ◆ Feel the association to the sensation in your body.

- ◆ Repeat the word out loud ten times.

- ◆ Again, feel the association to sensations in the body.

- ◆ Keep repeating the word in your mind for a minute.

- ◆ Feel the effect in the body.

- ◆ Separate the word into its two syllables – 'tin' and 'gling' – and put a one-second pause between the two syllables.

- ◆ Repeat this for a minute quietly in your mind and associate the 'tin' with arising sensations in the body and 'gling' with the sensations passing away. It can be any sensation, gross or subtle.

- ◆ Now drop the 'tin' and keep repeating 'gling'.

- ◆ Let the 'gling' and passing nature of the sensations become intimate with each other. This will enhance the perception of the passing of sensations and thus help them to be perceived as more and more subtle.

- ◆ Now let the awareness of passing be at the umbilicus region for a while. Then the heart region for a while, and finally the third ventricle for a while.

- ◆ Notice how this affects the whole body!

4.4 Arising and passing[20]

Silently observing potency, without any motor intent or excessive distraction, opens up a sense of arising and passing without the baggage of thought. When the mind settles even more, the sense of arising and passing can permeate the whole of our sensate world until passing and arising are the same! This is a revelational shift in perception. One might call it insight of the Planck scale, the quantum vacuum, or the zero-point field,[21] but again that would be limiting and 'thingifying' the perception, thus limiting the awareness of the potential unfolding scene. In this book, I will refer to this radical perspective as non-dual insight.[22]

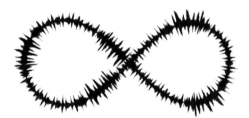

Figure 4.4: The tone of non-duality

See if you can notice the changing, tingling presence of one area on your body. Granted, as soon as we isolate the sensations, we limit them to space and time. So, notice how the rest of the body, and beyond, is resonating with this sense due to the very act of your perception at one point. Balanced awareness of one aspect of the body can provide the sense of potency. If this awareness perseveres for a length of time, without being distracted, the sense of emerging and passing can start to be appreciated.

The passing quality is the most difficult to understand and yet it is only by appreciating and feeling it that the insight of change can really be embodied. If passing, in this context, is understood merely by conceptualization then it will provide no felt-sense insight. In fact, the thought of passing can evoke a sense of sadness and even depression when it is not conjoined with insight. Conversely, when there is a felt-sense of passing, there can be a feeling of connection, love and beauty.

In yogic philosophy, the five phases/elements of nature consist of earth, water, fire, air and ether (space).[23] Each phase can be perceived as having particular qualities, such as temperature and transmutability for fire, cohesion for water, and so on. But it is the shared quality of their transitioning which provides insight. This transition is akin to the transition of winter to spring to summer, although this analogy can distract from the insight attained when one perceives the transition as passing, and understanding it as the fifth element. In other words, passing is space, space is potency. The quality of space holds potential for fresh arising (free from TI/ME). When this is truly felt and understood then arising and passing are no different. This felt-sense insight is what biodynamic craniosacral therapists call potency.

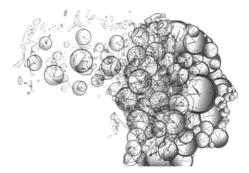

Figure 4.5: Passing TI/ME

4.5 Equanimity

The use of the word equanimity here is not the same as 'indifference'. It is the non-reactivity born from the insight of TI/ME passing.

The potent felt-sense quality of arising and passing is the same characteristic shared by any sensation, impression, memory or experience. However, with potency there is no interruption between arising and passing, caused by the contents of thought, and so arising and passing are felt as one.

If a thought-object is relished by the perceiver, the impression of sensation arising increases.[24] However, if there is sufficient aversion or fear towards a thought-object, it will evoke a dissociation from the arising sensation.[25] In both circumstances, the sense of arising is affected by an individual's conditioned tendency to either enhance the sensation[26] or dissociate from it.[27] In both circumstances, therefore, the perception of liking or disliking either reinforces the sensation or promotes a seeming unawareness of it, resulting in the felt-sense of passing away to reduce and the perception of potency to diminish. This presents an issue, as the perception of passing away will continue to reduce, to the point that potency is not noticed at all!

The passing characteristic of sensation, therefore, needs to be felt intimately for potency to be expressed fully and to enhance the insight of the nature of change. Insight of change is the awareness of arising and passing and understanding that they are not different – they are the same, much like the quantum particle and wave are in essence the same. If potency is not understood like this then potency becomes yet another 'thing' of the mind.

To recap: insight of the subtle nature of change is only truly understood with the sense of passing. This can be illustrated via the example of apnoea (cessation) during the breathing cycle. When the automatic nature of exhalation (passing) follows its course there is rarely a need to remember to breathe in, as it happens spontaneously following a short autonomic pause. But this is often not the case regarding inhalation (arising), as we can sometimes 'forget' to breathe out,[28] especially when we are caught in a cycle of anxiety and stress. This is because over-thinking and worrying, can inhibit the passive release of the diaphragm.[29]

In other words, potency gets stuck in a loop of continual arising without letting go, like the repetitive nature of a thought continuously repeating itself.

The sense of passing reveals an incredibly different scene to the one perceived and projected by thoughts associated to the sense of arising. That is because the essence of thought is now perceived, rather than its content. This profound perception is where the paradox of non-duality presents itself. In other words, arising and passing are perceived as not being different, in the same way nothing and everything or emptiness and fullness or stillness and dynamicness are the same, as there is no impression-based tendency separating them!

So, one either gets attached or dissociates to an impression (object) because of the reactive tendencies one has to the sense of arising. But we get released from these impression-based habits by the perceived sense of passing. The felt-sense of passing is the key to insight of change and understanding potency. This heals the chasm of duality[30] and results in a calm intensity of presence, joy, awe and thought fuelled by insight rather than reactive habit.

In the 1990s I got involved with, and smitten by, the martial art Brazilian jiu jitsu (BJJ) and a hybrid martial art called vale-tudo, which were starting to gain popularity around the globe. During a notable practice session bout, I remember grappling with a fellow who far outweighed me. I recall that he was quite intimidatory, simply because he was so skilled and agile. At one point I was pinned to the floor, on my back, with his full weight on my chest and his arms in a python-like choke hold around my neck. It seemed pointless to struggle, yet it somehow seemed unnecessary to tap out (give in). I yielded to the circumstance by sensing my whole body dissolve, but this was by no means a form of dissociating from my body, or the circumstance. My body was still there, but it was no longer limited by TI/ME. It was as if time no longer existed, at least in the self-referential chronological sense of that word, and space seemed to be unbounded – energy with infinite possibility. Moreover, I sensed the chap (who was trying to choke me out) dissolve too. He was still there, but he was now amorphous and his weight and strong arms were no longer an issue. I felt every idiosyncratic twitch and pulse in my opponent. The following moments were a bit of a blur, as my perception of time lagged behind what unfolded. But what I do recall is that my mind became empty of limits and my body became very full of energy. I moved so fast that the guy watching over us was later completely flummoxed as to what happened. I ended up putting the big dude into a BJJ 'check mate' position. This guy very rarely tapped out, because he usually didn't need to – but he did on that day. I was hugely struck by that event, and the insight of TI/ME passing has echoed in me ever since.

However, the deepest insight aspect I gleaned from that event was not so much the event itself, but what it led to, as I will now explain.

While I was getting immersed into the grappling arts I also started to investigate meditation, and became enamoured by the practice of Rinzai and Soto Zen. The practice provided such a balanced and resourcing way of 'seeing' things. It actually provided so much clarity for my inner world that it unveiled a deep inner conflict within me.

It was a conflict of where I should place my priorities in life and it began brewing heavily in my mind. Should I be investing my energy into building the skills to overpower another being, or should I dedicate my energy into investigating the source of harmony and insight?

A Zen teacher I encountered provided a profoundly helpful answer:

Learning the way of helping another surrender can provide insight by knowing that we ourselves must first surrender to a circumstance without losing contact with our source.

Yet awareness of death, in oneself, without imposing it on another, provides far more insight.

This is because death (passing) resides in each moment and, when realized, is itself an intimate aspect of life's expression. It is nature revealing its origin.

When there is enough awareness of this then there will be no need to invest energy into helping another surrender. You will now be far more interested in helping another to discover their original nature via your presence as a reference. This is also helping another to surrender, but your intent is now very different. Such intent will dissolve into and reveal the source far more readily, and with far greater impact – check it out.

Needless to say, I was considerably impacted and moved by what this teacher shared, so I was impelled to check it out.

In the context of this book we can interpret what the Zen teacher called death as TI/ME passing.

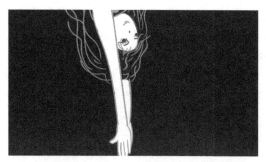

Figure 4.6: Diving into calm intensity

4.6 Curiosity

The calm yet intense interface which opens with the insight of TI/ME passing presents another quality other than equanimity. This quality is curiosity, which is often relatively veiled by TI/ME by the time we reach early adulthood. Curiosity is like the flow of a continually truly open question, open to receiving new and invigorating information without getting side-tracked by the clouding nature of old impressions.

The insight of TI/ME passing provides a receptivity which is fresh, new like the senses of a baby, ready to perceive the world without the baggage of analysis, judgement, formulation, labelling and so on. The END therapist, therefore, provides a *tabula rasa* mind as the underpinning ingredient to help promote relational touch, empty of TI/ME yet full of potential. It is the 'wow!' of genuine curiosity which encourages another person's system to reveal its subtle patterns.

WOW is actually an acronym I use to describe the 'wing opening wobble' of the sphenoid bone. Contact, with the thumbs or fingers, at the greater wings of the sphenoid on either side of the cranial vault, is extremely useful for encouraging a person's system to open to the relational field. However, if intention overtakes the insight of TI/ME passing, then this contact can become a pressure cooker hold for the client, as it is a very sensitive area to touch. It is, therefore, useful to contact this region in a fully present fashion and with minimal intention held in your system. When calm intensity is fully appreciated in the therapist with a wide perceptual field, the WOW often presents itself. It often demonstrates as a shimmer, wiggle or wobble of the client's head and neck as the passing of TI/ME starts to affect their nervous system, from being in a fragmented state to expressing as a whole – this is truly a wow moment.

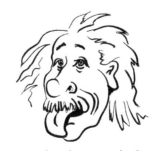

Figure 4.7: Einstein uncontrived curiosity

4.7 Ice, liquid, steam

A useful metaphor to help understand the passing of TI/ME is the process of ice (TI/ME) melting to liquid and liquid evaporating to steam. TI/ME only fully passes when it 'turns' into steam. The deepest impressions reside in the fluid field and perhaps these impressions are the ones which give us the unwavering sense of self-continuity like a stream of consciousness flowing through time.

Buddhist scholars refer to these deep impressions as *bhava sankharas*, impressions, which churn for long periods of time, like cyclical eddy currents in the stream of consciousness (*vinnana-sota*). These are generally the last patterns of experience to be perceived as passing (steam) and, if they are to be ascribed with a felt physical locality, they are mostly felt echoing in the organs, the deepest being the heart.

The tendencies (*vasanas*), built on these deep impressions, turn to steam much more readily and are usually the patterns providing the self with the sense of superficial separation and the basis for structuring mechanistic thought. Tendencies to like or dislike, want or not want, form the basis of our identity.

Each individual will have a particular propensity to notice the deeper patterns (*sankharas*). For some, this awareness might be developed to the point of being able to sense TI/ME passing at its subtlest. In such cases, the awareness of this subtlety will be via the auditory or visual sense. In both cases, they lead to what I call the 'gling of dissolution' or 'gleam of dissolution' (GOD), which opens to the vibration of sound, or light, untainted by TI/ME. They both resonate with the potency sense at the third ventricle of the brain and sinoatrial node of the heart, and open up to the wholistic interface of calm intensity, which will now be explained.

◆ Chapter 5 ◆

Entering Stillness

We cannot see our reflection in running water,
it is only in still water we can see.

TAOIST PROVERB

5.1 No permanent separate self

Many years ago, people thought that the world we live on was flat, with
a vast number believing it to be supported by four elephants standing
on a giant turtle.[1] This was the popular belief and was the prominent
one for not just centuries but millennia. Indeed, it was a simple one
and at the time would have seemed indisputable – in fact, a no-brainer!
Nonetheless, 2600 years ago, a philosopher called Anaximander evolved
the flat world perspective by postulating that the earth was actually a
cube, which is weird. Later a fellow called Parmenides proposed it was
a sphere, which complicated the perspective of things a little but it was
nevertheless accommodated by a few, and for these people it seemed
to make sense – phew!

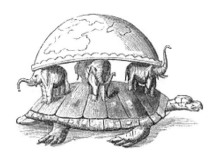

Figure 5.1: Turtle and elephants supporting the world

This was the beginning of the geocentric way of perceiving our place in the universe, which widened our perceptual understanding of where we were placed in relation to our environment, and, thus, our human-centric perspective developed another dimension.[2]

Then, a student of Plato's, called Aristotle, extended the geocentric theory which then took over from the old view. Needless to say, our place in the solar system shifted significantly as we re-orientated to our known universe. After this, a renaissance mathematician called Copernicus presented the heliocentric theory, which, as it turned out, appealed to a fair few people, despite later being banned by the church. Interestingly, an astronomer by the name of Aristarchus of Samos actually came up with the heliocentric model 18 centuries earlier! A wee while later, Galileo discovered our galaxy, the milky way, and, later still, the composer-astronomer, Herschel, expanded on this by estimating the position of our sun, hypothesizing that our sun was the centre of the disc-shaped milky way galaxy which resided in the centre of the universe. This was later disputed and overthrown by astronomers to become what is now known as the galactocentric model, which estimates that the centre of the galaxy is somewhere close to a star in the sagittarius constellation, nudging the centre of the universe over a bit. However, astronomers now know that this is also incorrect, as our galaxy itself is not the centre of the universe. Actually, it is difficult to say what is.

Why mention a bunch of ancient philosophers and astronomers from the past alongside the perspectives they held? Well it seems that society at large has adopted similar centric assumptions with regard to how we perceive ourselves in relation to the world. Our centra-phillic supposition comes from our inherent belief that we are separate individuals based on the impression that we are made from some permanent substance which is in the midst of everything else dancing around us. Yet, despite this perspective being a practical one (in many regards), it is also distorted, as will now be explained.

When Michelangelo was asked by the Pope about the secret of his genius, particularly how he carved the sculpture of David, his answer was: 'Simple, I just remove everything that is not David.' Let us borrow David from Michelangelo and use him as a metaphor to depict original nature. The stone, which is not David (i.e. delusion), falls away and only David (i.e. original nature) remains. Delusion is fragile, original nature is not. This approach is also called subtractive epistemology. Disconfirmation of what is held to be real (which could be delusion) is more rigorous than confirmation of the same. Disconfirmation in this regard continues until it cannot disconfirm anymore.[3] It will be found that this will only occur with the realization of non-duality. Nevertheless, stripping the unreal from the real takes time and effort.

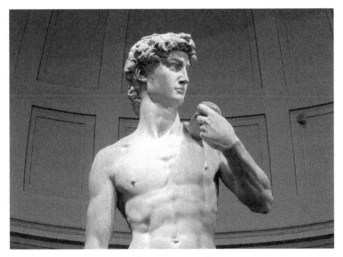

Figure 5.2: David

Waking to the reality does not strip away anything, it is merely a transmutation of perspective. Therefore, letting go of intention cannot be complete unless one wakes up to the reality of non-duality. The absolute nature of non-duality is incredibly simple, so simple that it can be very hard for the complexity of the mind to accept.

5.2 'No I', or 'I AM'?

The philosophical debate between the understanding of 'No I' and the understanding of 'I AM' has been going on for centuries. It is way beyond the scope of this book to cover such a huge debate. Nevertheless, for END therapists it can be useful to outline the benefits and drawbacks of perceiving these two seemingly opposite perspectives.

The only way to truly understand no independent, separate self

(No I) is to be aware of and realize the passing nature of TI/ME and body sensations, and be open to a quality free from TI/ME – the divisionless movement of arising and passing being the same. The quality free from TI/ME could be referred to as I AM, which is consciousness being self-aware via the 'mirror' of TI/ME passing to reveal its true nature.

Are these perspectives really different from one another? Yes, but only if the insight of TI/ME passing is absent. Insight, in this light, will not result in 'I' (ahamkara), superimposing itself as a higher self (atma) or supreme self (paramatma).

Without insight of TI/ME passing, identification will still be re-inforcing separation, despite how blissful and all-inclusive it might seem. There are a few teachers who seem to meet their audiences with insight, and it appears to be just a matter of semantics which differentiates No I from I AM. Yet there seem to be many teachers who do not. Be that as it may, it is interesting to note how much philosophy is often invested in defending each perspective.[4] Philosophy, without insight, will only increase the recalcitrance and identification to TI/ME and obscure insight with more and more complexity.[5] Nevertheless, dualistic simplicity can be equally problematic, as will now be explained.

5.3 Binary simple, complex and non-dual simple

Occam's Razor, or lex parsimoniae, is a philosophical principle which basically says that the more that assumptions are used to explain an occurrence, the more unlikely the explanation.

Our assumptions are born from concepts, and experience, which often miss out vital elements. Perspectives such as this are considered assumption heuristics[6] which promote a distorted impression of the world we perceive. However, that which we deem to be a simple explanation is still very likely to be complicated due to our conviction of our perception of the world,[7] which is actually an interpretation based on distorted impressions. We could consider this as 'binary simplicity', or BS.

To make matters worse, we often lead very complex lives, and yet many times we allude to the idea that we think simply. Thinking, by nature, is not simple. If there is thought then there is complication, based on the premise of there being a centre (me), 'me-centric'.

On hearing this, someone in the 'think simply group' might retort, 'Ah, but it is good to simplify things as much as possible whether there is the delusion of an identified centre or not.' Of course, this is often found to be true,[8] but it is useful not to further delude oneself into believing that this is the same simplicity we are discussing with non-doing.

Furthermore, the conceptual simplicity which nurtures complacency, but ignores gnawing unsatisfactoriness, could be likened to being happy driving round and round on a never-ending round-about without any exit or insight of what lays beyond it. It is like the simplicity and complacency a frog, born and living in a deep well, would use to describe its perspective of the ocean,[9] i.e. the water in the well is the perspective of an ocean to the frog. Whereas the idea of an ocean vast enough to fit more than a trillion frogs is a notion of utter poppycock.

The original Ch'an and Zen practices emphasized the importance of a student relinquishing the staleness of both complex and simple thinking,[10] in order to deepen their insight into the essence of non-doing. To facilitate this, the master will pose a conundrum for the student to solve. It may appear simple to solve and yet every answer the student offers is countered or rebuffed. The student will then sit with the riddle and the mind will delve deeper into a labyrinth of possibilities. Eventually the maze of possibilities becomes so complicated that the pressure causes the student to give up and let go of trying to work it out. It is in this moment there is the potential for insight.[11] The insight is born from the intensity and stimulus of thought building up until it is released and the awareness of its essence, rather than its content, is realized. The essence is our original nature, or what we refer to as dynamic stillness.

5.4 Accessing original nature

Engaged non-doing sounds easy to incorporate into a treatment session and it is not uncommon for us to think we just need to be still and quieten our minds and *voila* we are not doing anything. Yet, the reality of non-doing requires a great deal of inquiry, insight and practice, because non-doing is rarely embodied as a quality of insight and engagement. This means that there first needs to be an inquiry into the felt-sense of intention (doing) before there can be a real appreciation of non-doing. It can then be noticed that a non-reactive felt-sense inquiry into doing is non-doing! In other words, engaged non-doing means the end of both doing (intention) and lack of engagement.

A practitioner's awareness of and equanimity towards the sensations primed by attention, therefore, enables a calm intensity within oneself. This acts not only as a gateway to non-doing but also to realizing the source of the changing nature of body and mind – our original nature.

What is interesting, for us as END practitioners, is the surreptitious tendency for our intentions to seep into a session, despite our believing that we are not doing anything. The reason for this belief is that we don't realize that we are holding a desire for a particular outcome. This desire sets up the image of a goal which subsequently evokes a motor/'energetic' intention. In other words, our body will prime itself to try and 'do' something to help manifest the goal.

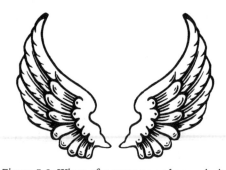

Figure 5.3: Wings of awareness and equanimity

Being aware of and equanimous towards the subconscious tendencies that support doing acts is an antidote to intention. Such awareness needs to be wholistic, as does equanimity to the changing nature of the sensations. This is a first step which aids in realizing the ephemeral nature of body sensations.

5.5 Flop, freeze, flight, friend and...freedom

Imagine a scenario where we encounter a grizzly bear while walking in the forest. If it is imminently close, our physiologic response will likely result in a dorsal vagal mediated dissociation from our bodily sensations and voluntary motor control. This is automatically established to save the sympathetic nervous system pumping unnecessary blood around the body. This flaccid 'flop' response is also an autonomic attempt to feign death in order to look like unpalatable carrion. Very clever, but if the grizzly is far enough away it is more likely that our body will freeze in a rigid manner, preventing movement, including digestive movements, and cut off all pheromonal production, while the mind whirs around postulating directions of escape. In this way, the bear is much less likely to see, hear or smell us. Again, very smart.

In yet another scenario, if we see the bear through a pair of binoculars, and the distance between us and the bear is sufficient, we might feel the surge of adrenaline be accepted by the major muscles of our legs and we will get the heck out of there. Yet, if we see that the closing figure is in fact not a bear at all but our tramping buddy whom we had lost on the trail, then we will probably fill up with ventral vagal ease and gravitate to their location.

These are the survival responses/states which can seep into our day-to-day interactions, even during time on our own. They blend into our association and identification with TI/ME and its resulting effect on our intentions to the point where it is rare for an hour to go by without one or more of these responses dictating our physiology. The heightened level of social engagement, encouraged by our ventral vagal system, is a goal of sorts, at least whenever the environment and company allow for it to be brought about without us being vulnerable to preventable harm, and our appraisal of any external danger is obviously important. However, dependence on another person's behaviour in order for us to be calm is not a fully conscious state. It is still a state at the mercy of TI/ME 'pulling the strings'.

Nevertheless, I would like to propose that there is another 'state', which is not dependent on another person, or people, presenting with particular patterns of behaviour. An inherent sense of safety which is calm yet intensely connected in all circumstances. A presence which is both free from, and in contact with, TI/ME. I call this 'calm intensity'.

Calm intensity is, therefore, being aware and non-reactive to sub-conscious tendencies, and is an antidote to TI/ME-derived intention. For this, an individual's awareness needs to be whole, as does one's equanimity towards the changing nature of the sensations in one's own body. This is a first step which aids in realizing the ephemeral nature of body sensations.

5.6 Calm intensity[12]

In this way, both subconscious and conscious intent unfold to be appreciated in a subtler and less identified manner, which opens up to an expression of sensation, de-clutched from the reactivity of like and dislike. This enables a transition from intent to an engaged felt-sense of TI/ME passing, which is the insight of change itself.[13] To describe the felt-sense quality of TI/ME passing and its wholistic representation is difficult, but one term stands out as adequate, albeit paradoxical, and that is the sense of 'calm intensity' (CI). Once there is sufficient CI then engaged/embodied non-doing (END) is the natural way of treating and any intentions are noticed as inhibitors to the potential for health expressing itself.

This way of treating is prorelational and expands on polyvagal theory.[14] Polyvagal theory proposes that the species of this planet have reached a phylogenic crescendo, as far as the ANS's ability to adapt in relation to interpersonal events is concerned. Polyvagal pioneer, Stephen Porges, calls this the social engagement response, or the 'friend response'. This is where a person has the capacity to be embodied and engaged while being calm (immobile or mobile while feeling safe).[15] Bodily cues and vocal tones offered by another are reciprocated and co-regulated by the recipient to provide balance and a felt-sense of being heard. The more trusting and sensitive a relational interaction gets, the more likely it will be for the communication to share subtle information.[16]

While a materialist's rationale for this sensitivity would be that the mirror neurones in one person (person a) are firing sufficiently to reciprocate and regulate with another (person b), the non-dualist would see this as the delusion of separation dissolving and providing an empowering reference for the essence of embodiment, rather than temporary relief from the feeling of disembodiment. Whichever perspective one takes, the realization of relationship in this regard is intense, which is not to say it is bad or good.[17] It can be so intense that person a might start to dissociate from their own sensations, if they are not accustomed to it.

In some circumstances 'social engagement' can transition into a theatric act, based on congenial expectations, by suppressing reactive tendencies to give the impression of social cordiality. Obviously, this belies the reality, and will undoubtedly form some sort of physiologic or psychologic inner conflict, but is obviously useful for social harmony. It is, therefore, useful to reaccess the suppressions at one's earliest convenience to prevent systemic disharmony.

However, if person a were to interact while aware of the intensity, and not react to it, then a deeper felt-sense empathy towards the other person will likely unfold, to the point at which we might now consider the relational interaction to be based on compassion.[18] This is because the felt-sense of relational communication now involves the insight of person a. In other words, person a is feeling for the other person by perceiving TI/ME passing.[19] Person b will feel this deeply, even if they are not aware of it. Therefore, person a is covertly helping to remind person b of the expression of health by perceiving the passing of TI/ME in their own body. To the materialist, this would be due to person a being sensitive to their sensations and helping person b by down-regulating their own systemic reactions. But to the non-dualist, this would-be awareness and equanimity are helping to lift the veil of delusion (duality) to reveal the dynamic stillness of wholeness and tacitly sharing the intimate vitality of this insight. It seems plausible that both perspectives are true.

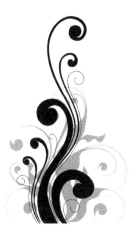

Figure 5.4: Koru (the Maori word for the shoots of the silver fern) – the potent stillness of unfolding

Coming back to the individual (person a), calm intensity is an engaged interlink hovering between the felt-sense of dynamic stillness and conditioned sensations.[20] It is, therefore, a link between duality and non-duality, the ultimate natural fulcrum.[21] Understanding and embodying the link between non-duality and duality is the standout feature in END therapy, and it is worth considering the impact the understanding has on our confidence in this therapy. With such understanding we will find that comparing this approach with other models of therapy, based on intending to change something, is pointless as we are relinquishing intention itself. Moreover, the rationale underpinning this therapy can be understood as being beyond any unfelt abstract explanations such as calling it a placebo response, as will be discussed in the next section.

If research is required to add heady credibility to the 'existence' of this vibrational interface (CI), then the researcher has already asserted TI/ME to try and measure the passing of TI/ME – how unfortunate. For example, if someone were to substitute the felt-sense of calm intensity with a quantifiable measurement by placing a few electroencephalogram leads on a person's skull, producing a graph of ascending and descending lines, then TI/ME would be trying to make 'known' the frequency of the universe – instead of being it.

Some may access the felt-sense insight of TI/ME passing by 'only seeing' or 'only hearing'.[22] Whatever sense door is used it will relay as a vibration throughout and around the body. This is the interface of calm intensity. When including another person, or people, this calm intensity insight fuels loving kindness – otherwise known as *metta*.

5.7 Beyond the placebo

Dr Herbert Benson is the cardiologist who coined the phrase 'remembered wellness', which provided a positive spin on the placebo effect and countered the negative connotations the word received from pharmaceutical research. Benson's interpretation enables an empowering perspective for many people, helping them to resource their well-being by positively thinking about their potential and inherent health. By recalling the wellness endowed within themselves, Benson demonstrated that individuals become less dependent on external input, and/ or intervention, to improve their health.

Dr Joe Dispenza[23] has expanded on the practical application of remembered wellness by prompting a popular contemporary movement which fosters the perspective that we *are* the placebo in and of ourselves. He goes on to encourage practising certain meditation techniques that help the mind to relinquish its habit of collapsing into set patterns and as a result 'making' our mind matter, literally.

Nevertheless, as relatively useful as Benson's and Dispenza's perspectives and approaches may be, there is an inherent problem with them. That is that the application of any technique is dependent on the content of thought, and if the content of thought is not 'seen' for what it is (duality) then what is in this case called positive (remembered wellness) will inevitably manifest its opposite (remembered unwellness). To illustrate: when one relishes the reactive tendency (preference) to surround and imbibe oneself with objects, events, substances and so on, which evoke pleasant sensations, this tendency will simultaneously weaken equanimity towards those objects, events, relationships, substances which evoke unpleasant sensations and, therefore, the 'positive' lowers the threshold for reacting with aversion towards the 'negative' (that which is not preferred).

Dispenza seems to already know this but he circumvents the issue by implying that via meditation on 'no-thing', 'no-time' and 'no-self' (conceptual non-duality, rather than felt-sense non-duality) the content of thought will be filtered of its negativity. This is simply a superficial band-aid to cover that which is subjectively not liked in order to elevate that which is liked. The default mode network[24] of the brain is, therefore, still pulling the strings. The eventual outcome, based on the desire to be free of the unpleasant, becomes a major impediment to perceiving the full array of felt-sense expressions and will inevitably lead to potential limitation of awareness (relative dissociation), and reduced equanimity, towards anything perceived as negative. So, in effect, such 'positive'-inducing techniques will enhance the shadow, due to favouring the light. This is like trimming the branches of suffering while nourishing the roots.

If a therapist comes from such preferential perspective then their felt-sense awareness of the inherently changing nature of physiology will be stymied. This does not mean that Dispenza is wrong, from a conceptual perspective, but if no-thing, no-time and no-self is not a felt-sense insight then the intention (the goal) will merely be veiling the 'thing', 'time' and 'self' with the impression of not being an object, time or self, rather than realizing the felt-sense reality of no-thing, no-time and no-self.

The reason for the effectiveness of END therapy, therefore, is not merely the positive perspective of the placebo response; its major benefit resides beyond this in the source of awareness and equanimity and does not require 'making' anything into matter. Bearing this in mind, let us look into how we can better understand and practise END, in order to optimize being in touch with 'the source' rather than getting something from it.

Q: If any manipulation, 'making', method, process or technique involves intent, how do we approach this?

A: Read on.

◆ Chapter 6 ◆

Calm In-10-City

It is too clear and so it is hard to see.

A fool once searched for a fire with a lighted lantern. Had he known what fire was, he could have cooked his rice much sooner.

EKAI, THE GATELESS GATE

6.1 The ten characteristics of a 'city' with no gate

When we become aware of the veil[1] obscuring our original nature, a quality exposes itself, if only for a fraction of a second. It reveals a 'city'[2] of intense potency, which has the capacity for providing invaluable insight. It is difficult to explain this insight without using inappropriate words. To understand its paradoxical and unseparated nature the reader needs to frequently hone in to the felt-sense of their ever-changing body sensations. Sensing the arising and passing nature of the sensations of your own body, as you read through the rest of this chapter, has the potential to open insight rather than mere knowledge.

Skilful navigation from intent to non-doing can be dissected into ten essential characteristics which an END therapist may notice and gain momentum from. The crescendo of these is felt as a wholistic calm intensity, which acts as a felt-sense interface between TI/ME (duality) and dynamic stillness (non-duality). Together these characteristics are referred to as 'calm in-10-city'[3] (CITC).

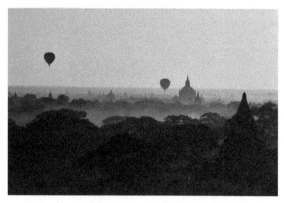

Figure 6.1: Calm in-10-city (the city of insight)

Note that the CITC characteristics are explained at various points in this book, and not necessarily in the following order.

Qualities of calm in-10-city[4]

1. **Attention:** Specific Area of Sensation Awareness (SASA); awareness stretching itself to sense TI/ME passing.

2. **Passing:** Settling; felt-sense of TI/ME dissolving; increases equanimity.

3. **Awareness and equanimity:** 1 and 2; state of balanced awareness.

4. **Calm intensity:** 1, 2 and 3; wholistic perception; TI/ME dissolution to sense fluids (mind's interpretation = 'mid-tide'); TI/ME dissolution to sense potency (mind's interpretation = 'long-tide').

5. **Insight:** 1, 2, 3 and 4; felt-sense understanding of TI/ME passing, no-thing, no-time, no-self.

6. **Dynamic stillness:** 1, 2, 3, 4 and 5; arising is passing; divisionless movement; original nature.

7. **Primal midline (*li*[5]):** 1, 2, 3, 4, 5 and 6; self born from insight and the experiencing of dynamic stillness.

8. **Felt-sense connection:** 1, 2, 3, 4, 5, 6 and 7; insight of feeling the

sensations and TI/ME of 'another', free from misperception of being merged.

9. **Transmutation:** Shift and reorganization occurring in the client's system with integration of the aforementioned characteristics.

10. **Loving appreciation:** Thoughts and feelings born from insight.

Despite these qualities being labelled and separated for intellectual understanding, it is valuable to consider that each one contains the essence of all the others. Perhaps more importantly, each quality comes to fruition by way of effortless effort, resulting in a midline of 'knowing' untainted by the known. It is, therefore, not so much a process as it is an understanding – the understanding of original nature navigating its way back to itself.

Undivided, the felt-sense of these qualities can be perceived as both intensely vibrant and peacefully calm. Furthermore, and perhaps the most radical thing to appreciate about the CITC characteristics, is that together they engender a sense which acts as an interface between the perception of duality (relative perception) and the insight of non-duality (absolute awareness).

How can this be possible?

To help answer this it is important to accrue some relevant experiential exercise mileage. Retreat-style meditation courses such as the renowned S.N. Goenka Vipassana[6] silent retreats are a relevant and very useful endeavour as they put at least a 90 per cent emphasis on the practice of experiencing reality as it is (*yatha bhuta*), rather than some intentionally formulated experience,[7] and only about 10 per cent on theory. From a therapeutic bodywork perspective, the global Body Intelligence[8] courses are a good example, as they place considerable importance on the need to explore the real-time expressions of the body rather than forming constructs and imaginations based on theory. However, neither of these courses jettisons the need for theory as an orientation tool for the mind. It is the predominance of unimagined sensation-based practice (*pati-pati*), over theory (*paryati*), which makes the success of these courses stand out.

When calm intensity is genuinely felt for what it is then any physiology theory, such as embryology (which we may have sweated over for years), will now become understandable and alive as a tone of felt-sense body expression. Let's face it, an embryo doesn't need to have an ability to theoretically dissect itself to access the expression of its own health because the calm intensity of wholeness is enough – more than enough.

The CITC characteristics will be explored in detail later in this book to help orient the reader to relevant experiential practices. They will also be simplified in other ways for those requiring a more palatable understanding.

6.2 Non-doing versus progressive approach

Rather than these ten qualities being effortlessly applied, they can also be strived for via various progressive methods. However, the very striving for these qualities can lead to further obscuration by TI/ME. The reason for this is because when there is striving there is a goal, and the nature of a goal invokes a separation between the striver (impression of self) and the object strived for (projected by thought, fuelled by TI/ME). If there is a separation between the impression of self and thought then the ten qualities become 'perfections', which require attention to attain, but often surreptitiously incorporate identification, and of course involve time to achieve. They are, nonetheless, meritworthy aspirations which may help order and relax the mind, if truly embodied. These perfections, often mentioned in Buddhist literature, are as follows: 1) Generosity, 2) Wisdom, 3) Moral conduct, 4) Patience, 5) Equanimity, 6) Determination, 7) Truthfulness, 8) Energy, 9) Renunciation, 10) Loving kindness.

Both non-doing and progressive approaches can be useful to enable and enhance a calm mind conducive for concentration. Nevertheless, an approach freed from intention is the only approach that will provide insight of TI/ME passing and into the divisionless movement of dynamic stillness. The reason for this is that one needs to touch the unlimited with the unlimited because only the unlimited knows the unlimited. Similarly, only the limited can only know the limited. Intention is always finite as its focus excludes the felt-sense of infinite potential. Realizing this helps one understand how an appropriate intention can be when used as a platform to augment enough attention to access calm intensity. Embodiment of calm intensity acts as an interface between the infinite and the finite, enough for a client to feel met, and provided with a reference to something beyond typical reactive touch. It is a fearless form of communication. At some point, this communication results in a client feeling able to orientate awareness to their own body from a fearless, wholistic felt-sense perspective.

So, if intention continues beyond its purpose as an access platform, and becomes a goal-driven approach, it limits potential and possibilities and therefore limits the expression of health. It is useful to remember this.

◆ EXPERIENTIAL EXERCISE 8

Calm in-10-city

◆ Bring your awareness to anywhere on your body which resonates with you at this moment.

◆ Notice you are definitely aware of this region of your body.

◆ It might be that you can discern that there is a diffuse boundary, like the diffuse peripheral vision of your eyesight when focusing on an object.

◆ Let awareness of the diffuse boundary gain prominence, and let the definite awareness of the known region you have become aware of fade.

◆ Now invite equanimity to this diffuse attention. In other words, notice the desire to be aware of another area, or the arising thought, or the sensation which is now pulling your attention away.

◆ Persevere with the awareness of this diffuse boundary, as it will likely widen and enable more awareness of the subtle nature of the sensations beyond this. The subtle sensations may also start to transform the solid perception of the area you were originally focused on so that the inner and outer environment are no longer completely separate.

◆ You may notice a transmutation of perspective unfold as the solid becomes more and more subtle. This engenders a felt-sense insight of TI/ME passing, which diminishes the impression of being separate from 'objects'.

◆ With such insight there is often a pervading sense of calmness, which isn't separate from a sense of aliveness/intensity.

◆ From here, see if you are naturally aware of your primal midline, potency, fluids and tissues.

◆ The spectral integration of realizing this calm intensity is free from intent and therefore full of fearless potential/health.

CLINICAL NOTE

When a practitioner keeps noticing and acknowledging the characteristics inherent with calm in-10-city, then insight of arising and passing will get clearer and clearer, until it reaches a point whereby there is no need to continue noticing. This is because 'you', your arising, passing and awareness, are now the same.

When this point is reached, engaged non-doing takes care of itself, as the impetus of no intention will enable the relevant perceptual field needed (for the system of the presenting client) and bring clarity to the practitioner as a primal midline of sensations. This is non-doing.

However, before we can immerse ourselves in the slipstream of non-doing, we must first access it.

Chapter 7

Access Attention

Attention leads to immortality. Carelessness leads to death. Those who pay attention will not die, while the careless are as good as dead already.

GAUTAMA THE BUDDHA (FROM THE DHAMMAPADA)

7.1 Access attention

Access attention is a unique form of focus which enhances the state of balanced awareness in a therapist in order to meet a client with embodied presence. Access attention is awareness honed in on a specific focal area of sensations on the body. This honing-in includes an element of tension, because attention is awareness collapsing from wholeness of the particular, which also accommodates TI/ME.

TI/ME fuels intention, so there will be a meeting of 'waves', whereby awareness meets intention. Sustained attention of this meeting leads to non-doing, which is the effortless effort of witnessing TI/ME, including intention, pass. As a result, attention also returns to its origin (awareness) and the tension of focus turns into awareness of the whole of the body and beyond the boundaries of what is perceived by TI/ME as a body.

This form of attention, however, is often stymied by the phrenetic nature of the monkey mind[1] (TI/ME). In other words, the waves clash. It is, therefore, advantageous to incorporate methods that help to settle the mind and not expect the mind to automatically sink into a state of balanced awareness.

A good way to achieve this, if required, is to understand, interpret[2] and practise the relevant aspects of the eight limbs (supporting components) of *raja* yoga[3]: the first two components, moral conduct and self discipline (*yama* and *niyama*), are practices which are not within the scope of this book to outline or discuss at any length. While some consider these limbs vital foundations for a deepening into the other limbs, others believe that they grow naturally as the other limbs are developing. There are even some who maintain that identifying with these first two limbs can prevent real understanding (insight) of the later limbs. Suffice to say that not intending to harm[4] (including oneself), and to discipline oneself to return to the subtle expression of nature when the mind is getting taken over by TI/ME, are adequate foundations for the balanced hypertrophy of the other limbs.[5]

The *raja* yoga perspective of posture and physiologic awareness (*asana*) is very useful for the END practitioner to understand, practise and feel. For example, spinal extension postures are useful to counter the mind caught by lethargy. If one gets used to occasionally adopting and sustaining extension postures with felt-sense awareness, then the body will get a boost. A slight backward bend of a couple of centimetres will be enough to wake the system up and encourage access attention, if needed. Conversely, if the practitioner's mind is excessively agitated, then forward spine curling helps it to calm.[6] Again, if we are well versed with the felt-sense effects of this body posture, then only a slight movement into it, for a brief period of time, is sufficient to pacify the mind.

If a person's mind is neither sleepy or agitated, but is not sensitive to the subtle sensations of their body, then rotation postures are a fantastic way to get a sense of the body fluids,[7] and a sense of opening. Inversions provide a sense of potency ascending (i.e. a sense of one's midline), slowing down and expansiveness. One might comment on the fact that while rotations would be easy to incorporate into the beginning of a treatment session, without the client realizing, inversions would be a bit more obvious. This is true, but not necessarily the case before touching the client. If I ever feel that my sense of midline is too distant for access attention then I bow for a short period (if it doesn't seem that it will freak out the client) or I just imagine doing a headstand. That is often all that is needed to remind the system of its intelligence.

Certain body gestures (*mudras*) and eye-gazing positions (*drishtis*) can also be used to achieve similar benefits to help balance the mind ready for access attention.

Breath-work is an aspect of postural and physiologic awareness and is extremely useful for balancing the mind ready for access attention, but it is often misinterpreted as the predominant feature of the fourth limb of yoga, awareness of the natural breath (*pran-ayama*) (Clarke, 2011).

Awareness of respiratory inhalation (*puraka*) can invigorate a tired mind, whereas awareness of exhalation (*rechaka*) can calm a busy mind. Similarly, brief retention of the breath at the end of exhalation (*bahya kumbhaka*) can promote a sense of the body fluids and bionimbus, whereas brief retention at the end of the in-breath (*antar kumbhaka*) can evoke a sense of potency rising. When a therapist is well acquainted with the felt-sense effects of such *asana* then access attention at specific areas becomes easy.

It is useful to become familiar with specific areas on your own body which have a particular sensitivity. These regions vary from person to person. Still, there are areas of heightened sensitivity which are fairly common and these will be outlined in this chapter. Once recognized, these specific regions of sensitivity can be used for initial access attention.

If sensations are not felt at the specific area of choice then gazing at a visible area or noticing the sound in the area can replace the felt-sense to begin with. For example, if a practitioner is feeling low or fatigued, then gazing at the curved area between the eyebrows[8] for a few minutes can help revitalize the system. If the therapist is feeling activated and finding it difficult to concentrate, then gazing at the nose tip[9] can help balance the mind. After a few minutes of gazing, awareness should be encouraged to notice the felt-sense of either the area which has been gazed on, or any other area which may have opened up.

The acronym SASA[10] stands for Specific Area of Sensation Awareness. There are many areas on the body where a practitioner can place attention, such as the area below the navel,[11] or the xiphoid process,[12] or the philtrum of the upper lip. Or, more subtly, the retina of the eye, the tympanic membrane of the ear, the epithelial cilia of the nose and so on.

These areas help the practitioner to become aware of a finite space within which sensations arise. For example, sensations can be felt at the area below the navel, where the abdomen is moving due to the breath, or at the pulse of the aorta close to the left-hand side of the navel. Sometimes it can be felt by feeling the 'hum' at the xiphisternum. During this attentive focus a felt-sense awareness of the gut space can open up.[13]

The heart space[14] can be accessed most easily at the manubrial notch, again initially via awareness of the movement of the natural breath, or the carotid pulse beat.

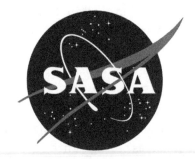

Figure 7.1: Specific Area of Sensation Awareness

7.2 Philtrum

The philtrum of the upper lip is quite unique, in that it is an area where we can feel the external touch of the breath on the skin, as well as subtle artery pulses. The awareness of the natural breath in this way is in fact the fourth limb of yoga, *pran-ayama*.[15] This awareness enables a sense of opening to both the space of the cranium[16] and the skin as a whole organ. Another interesting feature, and perhaps function, is the ability it has to scoop and funnel[17] airborne pheromones to be sensed by the vomeronasal organ. Despite this organ almost disappearing in humans, it has been found to be more developed in some people. The philtrum, therefore, is a useful access point to help a practitioner (and, in relevant circumstances, the client) to feel embodied and aware of the spaces of the body.

If none of the example access points provide access, then try somewhere else. For instance, place attention at one of the *chakras* regions (see Glossary) but try to apply the same principles. Every individual will have a different propensity for enabling access at different regions of the body. Inquire, explore – and ease into it for yourself to find out your own propensity.

7.3 Breath-fast, lung-ch and su-purrr

The awareness of the breath touching the skin at this highly sensitive area below the nose is enhanced when we subtly orchestrate the shortening of our own breath (to reach the respiratory tidal volume (TV) or less).[18] When we comfortably limit the length of our breath, the capillaries throughout the body dilate and the sensitivity of our tissues increases. Every now and then it might feel necessary to breathe in more deeply, and this could be referred to as time for 'lung-ch'. One or two deeper breaths are generally all that are needed before returning to 'breath-fast'. The felt-sense effect following a few minutes of this breath-work is a subtle wholistic tingling/purr throughout the body. The more pervasive this felt-sense becomes, the less intention to limit the breath that is needed[19] – in this case you can skip lung-ch and enjoy su-purrr.

◆ EXPERIENTIAL EXERCISE 9

Awareness mealtimes
Breath-fast

Being aware of the natural breath while in a calm unprovocative environment generally provides the catalyst for a natural tapering off of the breath. The body and mind settle enough for the breath to shorten. However, this effect can sometimes be established sooner if there is a gentle intention to limit the inhalation (very slightly). After practising this breath-fast for a minute or two, the body will automatically adapt by dilating the capillaries to enable more gaseous exchange to and from the tissues. Regular practice of breath-fasting will increase the plasticity of the vascular response.[20] The duration of practice can be anywhere from two minutes to two hours (or longer). The more regularly this is practised, the more adaptable the body is likely to become.

Lung-ch

This part of the practice acknowledges the need for taking a deeper breath at various points. Initially it may be that a deep breath is required every 30 seconds. However, with regular practice you may notice the ability to extend the duration of not needing to breathe deeply.

Su-purrr

The most important aspect of this exercise, at least as far as it is related to END therapy, is the awareness of the subtle sensations which show themselves during and following the practice. Often the sensations will be felt as a deep groundswell of subtle potency often mimicking the felt-sense of the vibration of a cat's purr when it is relaxed on your lap.

Acknowledging these subtle sensations is one of the best ways to become aware of TI/ME passing without getting lost in imagination.

7.4 Sensory balance

Another useful aspect of access attention is that it can help balance the sensory component of the cranial nerves.

If we can incorporate attention,[21] equanimity and insight[22] in certain areas then the intention we used initially to focus will dissipate, along with the reactions bound to these areas. In this way, the sensations will become subtler and the awareness of the rest of the body greater.

It is useful to become familiar with the location of these and other regions of the body. Reviewing anatomy and physiology images, even if the theory is not delved into that deeply, can be useful to access deeper felt-sense awareness. This is so for two main reasons: one that it enables the mind to be more familiar with the body, so that if the therapist gets consumed by TI/ME before or during a treatment session, then it can help her or him to orientate back to the present moment of the body (the therapist's body).

The second reason is that when we are aware of a specific area of the body, in a non-doing way, it starts to reveal the essential nature of the subtle expressions in the rest of the mind-body.

Awareness in this way is the fifth limb of yoga (*pratyahara*) and sustaining the awareness (attention) is the sixth limb of yoga (*dharana*), which opens to the insight of TI/ME passing (calm intensity) which is the seventh limb of yoga (*dhyana*). It is very common for people to mistake *dhyana* for body dissociation/transcendence, whereas insight of arising and passing is the primary quality of *dhyana*. This means one is both in touch with the manifest and the unmanifest.

7.5 Subtle sense awareness

There are other access points which are significantly more subtle than the ones mentioned. Yet each individual will be able to access the subtlety of these points with differing success. For example, some might have a powerful predisposition to resonate with the subtlety of vision consciousness. This can result in the access point being perceived as white light, which is a potent awareness of the third ventricle opening the awareness of the whole body. Others might have a subtle awareness of auditory consciousness, which is often perceived as a sound that can't be labelled and can at times seem as if it is sound originating from outside but is in fact the internal, high-pitched and potent tone of the central nervous system (a distinctively different sound from a medically diagnosed inner ear condition). It is actually the epicentre of the brain, the silent space of the ventricles, that 'listen' (access attention) to the sound.

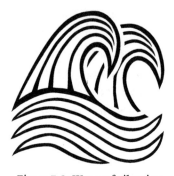

Figure 7.2: Waves of vibration

It is good here to discover whether you have a propensity to one of the sense consciousness vibrations. If, after some time of checking out if there is access to subtle light or sound, and it becomes apparent that the sense consciousness is not present, then it is useful to develop the touch awareness of an isolated area of the body instead. It can take an extremely long time to access the subtle awareness of vision and auditory consciousness if it is not a natural propensity for the individual. The awareness of sensations arising and passing on one area of the body is perfectly sufficient for opening to calm intensity, so don't get side-tracked.

A point of caution for those who do have a propensity to open to the third ventricle: if you establish a one-pointed attention here (*cittass-ekaggata*) then remember not to get stuck here as if the body does not exist. Such a state serves no purpose for a body therapist. When you include the subtle and potent awareness of your body then you will be treating from a non-reactive calm intensity and the client's system will feel met and safe to express itself, sometimes at great depth.

7.6 Access to natural fulcrum expression

When there is a natural relaxation of the access point attention, TI/ME dissolves and sinks back into its source. Generally, the body then starts to reveal itself in a different way as it turns to equanimity and insight (calm intensity).

At first, the body will reveal various patterns of experience and perhaps even disclose the undulating pattern(s) of its journey. These patterns may be brief or prolonged, yet with equanimity it doesn't matter.

Usually, attention promoting a specific point of sensation awareness unearths patterns of experience which are often short lived, as the insight of arising and passing is too great for such reactions to persist. Moreover, the state of balanced awareness is no longer perceived by the therapist as a mere 'state', as it is now imbued with insight, providing awareness of 'intention' beyond TI/ME, i.e. 'ground intention'.

After access attention has been sustained for a while, the body's deep natural fulcrums start to open and express themselves. These natural fulcrums are embryologic expressions, acting as motile pivots from within one of the four chambers of each of the three major cavities[23] – the lamina terminalis (anterior portion of the third brain chamber), the right roof of the right heart atrium (tissue supporting the sinoatrial node – first heart chamber) and the mesenteric attachment to the distal median ileum (*tan tien* – third gut-tube chamber).

As the therapist's equanimity deepens, intention dissipates and sustained attention increases, another quality presents itself: the sense spaciousness will expand beyond the limits of cavity separation. This quality of spaciousness can also be felt when a practitioner is caught in the 'grey zone', albeit with one vital quality missing – insight. Awareness of arising and passing is the defining quality which distinguishes insight from dissociation. This is important for a therapist to suss out, as it is the make or break in realizing the health-promoting capacity of calm intensity,[24] or getting carried away by the pleasant nature of a tide-like feeling.

Access attention is, therefore, an ignition to start the non-doing approach, at least at first. Once non-doing is humming it will become clear that it is the only 'way' to meet and greet 'ground intent', also known as original nature.

◆ EXPERIENTIAL EXERCISE 10A

SASA (we have lift off)
Vedana dharana

- ◆ Acquire a feather from inside a pillow, or use a piece of loose cotton wool.

- ◆ Attach it to the bottom of your philtrum (upper lip under nose tip) with a tiny piece of sticky tape.

- ◆ Sit comfortably and notice the breath.

- ◆ Try not to move the feather or cotton wool with your breath.

- ◆ Focus on this point of the body, making sure not to move the feather/cotton wool. Your breath is the only intention needed; awareness will enable the rest.

- ◆ Notice the touch of the breath as it touches the skin of the philtrum – this is not intent, it is awareness. The focus and subtle breathing pattern is intent in the form of the slightest control and attention (stretched awareness on an object).

- ◆ The intent will start to be replaced with mere awareness as the touch of the breath reveals the subtler sensations.

- ◆ Notice how this acts as a door to opening up to the subtle sensations of the rest of the body.

- ◆ Is there an appreciation of the A+P of these sensations?

- ◆ Open up to the natural fulcrums of the body.

- ◆ Let the cavities demonstrate and declare space.

- ◆ We are now ready to open up to perceptual fields with insight.

◆ EXPERIENTIAL EXERCISE 10B (PROGRESSION)

Dissolving into the source
Neti neti

- ◆ Sit in a comfortable position.

- ◆ Let awareness sink back to its source.

- ◆ Awareness of awareness being aware.

- ◆ Neither this, neither that.

- ◆ Notice that thought, any thought, is its source (not the impression of the object).

- ◆ Notice that sight, sound, touch, smell, taste is this source (not the impression of the object).

- ◆ Notice that all feelings and sensations are this source (not the impression of the object).

- ◆ Realize this is insight.

- ◆ Calm intensity is the felt-sense of this insight.

- ◆ Calm intensity touches the world of duality with the insight of non-duality (tantra).

NB: SASA is the bottom-to-top approach (*avidya* to *vidya*), whereas DITS is the top-to-integration approach (*vedanta* to *tantra*).

◆ Chapter 8 ◆

Insight Field

I went to the woods because I wished to live deliberately, to front only the essential facts of life, and see if I could not learn what it had to teach, and not, when I came to die, discover that I had not lived.

HENRY DAVID THOREAU

8.1 It is 'This'

Now that we have become aware of the type of intention which does not come from TI/ME, we can re-familiarize ourselves with the perceptual fields. The wider the perceptual field, the easier it is to appreciate the perceptual fields in the whole spectrum of awareness. When there is the perception of a wide field, with insight, it can be realized that it was actually already 'there'. That means no intent is needed to 'go out there'. We are already there (while being here), arising and passing (*avyaktam*) are everywhere. We are inherently that same expression of nature – the essence of 'it' is 'This'.

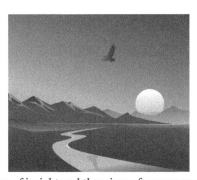

Figure 8.1: Moon of insight and the wings of awareness and equanimity

I vividly recall talking to my friend Jolyen after school one day. We were both about eight years old. Spontaneously one of us innocently asked out loud: 'Where does space end?' We were both quiet for a while and tingled with subtle sensations in the silence of the vast unanswerable question. TI/ME was not interrupting or trying to repeat the sensations, at least for a few moments, and 'the infinite' was not limited by it. In other words, the 'answer' was provided by sensation, not by thought.

Until 'This' is realized the perception of matter can be the only rational explanation for consciousness. Yet when 'This' vibrates, without limits, then TI/ME is perceived as passing in each moment, resulting in consciousness itself being reflected. In other words, consciousness is already 'everything' and 'nothing', the vibration of the infinite and the eternal. The icing on the cake comes with the realization of TI/ME passing, which amplifies the awareness of awareness being omnipresent and omnipotent – it is 'This'.

8.2 Present in all fields

The huge benefit with being aware and understanding 'This' is that we are present in the whole array of perceptual fields and, therefore, do not need to do anything to bring them about. This is useful, as we no longer need to intentionally narrow or widen our perpetual field to accomodate a client's perpetual inclination. The accomodation happens naturally. In other words, if we notice the expression of arising and passing in all fields, then the ground intent[1] (*tanmatra*) takes care of the relational requirements – 'This' is realized as the essence of what is commonly perceived as 'That'.[2]

◆ EXPERIENTIAL EXERCISE 11

Perceptive fields
Maha akasha vidya

- ◆ Be present with the awareness of the fluid expression and space in your body.

- ◆ Open to the wide perceptual field.

- ◆ Wonder to yourself: 'Was it already there?'

- ◆ Perhaps ask: 'Was I distracted from realizing the wide perceptual field?'

- ◆ The awareness of the wide perceptual field enables potency to take centre stage.

- ◆ Notice whether the potency starts to form the rhythmic theme of a slow gentle tide.

- ◆ Is there A+P insight with this theme?

- ◆ If there is, it is probable that you are aware of something deeper than the long tide – you are aware of calm intensity.

- ◆ This is the gateway to dynamic stillness, as well as being the gateway for ground intent.

- ◆ From here, enter the 'ease'.[3]

- ◆ This is the essence of our practice as END therapists – it is non-doing!

Setting up like this prior to and during treatment is deeply enhancing for a therapist's understanding, contact and effect on the client's system. It is useful to know that 'prior to treatment' does not just mean a few minutes before you make contact with a client. It means honing your awareness through practice at home and in daily life outside the clinic, at regular intervals.

8.3 Felt-sense of another

Prior to the interpretation of sensory input, for example the image of an object entering our eye sense door, we are somehow involved with it. This act of involvement is the moment of intimate experiencing, or presence. In other words, for a moment we are inseparably entangled with what is perceived, prior to it taking shape as an object.[4] Awareness of this entanglement is the perception of non-dual relationship, which the conditioned mind is not privy to because of its reliance on duality shaping the known world.

So, in the case of a conditioned mind, the moment of experiencing is clouded by what is already known, which fragments experiencing (presence) into experience (past). The experience is then contained in a package we call memory, which acts to support the notion of being separate yet related to the experience. Consequentially, the past justifies our position as 'me' being at the centre of experience, which reinforces the impression of being a separate, permanent self capable of changing circumstances in the present to promote an optimal future.

Despite such a view being very useful for practical orientation, including the manipulation of our environment, it is also skewed as it has suppressed the relational felt-sense of entanglement, resulting in assumptions fuelling what we 'know' rather than insight expanding what we feel.[5]

We are, therefore, missing a fundamental aspect of perception which, if acknowledged, could provide a greater sense of involvement to our infinite environment, and perceive a presence free of the known world, but not divorced from it.

Such presence is the awareness of TI/ME's absence, rather than the absence of awareness.[6] This is a very simple experiential 'model' which replaces the 'known' quagmire, whether formulated by the idealistic or materialistic philosophies of the world,[7] with insight – the most profound insight being awareness of the passing of TI/ME (psychologic time; past/future).

To provide further clarity let's postulate another perspective:

Q: What if we were to perceive ourselves as change itself?

At the macroscopic level, it is not so hard to conceptualize ourselves as constantly changing, as we reflect on the image we have of ourselves morphing over time in size, shape and weight and so on. But at the microscopic level, we need to replace conceptualization with awareness of the changing nature of our sensations. They cannot be felt in the past, they can only be felt in the present.

The felt-sense perception of changing sensations in our body starts to dissolve our recalcitrant centre-based perspective. Therefore, the centre-based perspective no longer holds as much relevance, because the past cannot infiltrate the intimate perception of feeling the changing nature of sensations.

By being aware of the delusive nature of identification, we find that the components of psychologic time is revealed. These components are reactive tendencies, imprinted impressions and identification to these, subconscious memories, expectations and patterns of experience (TI/ME), and are the catalysts for intention.

Therefore, it is beneficial to glean a non-centric perspective in the therapeutic setting to help the therapist to be present with the reality of what is unfolding, free from the encumbering reactivity of TI/ME.

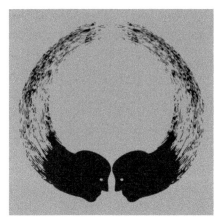

Figure 8.2: Origin to entanglement to insight

The huge therapeutic benefit deriving from this is that the therapist will, at times, feel certain patterns of the client expressing in their own body (the therapist's) and, with the insight of TI/ME passing, the patterns will transmute. For example, the therapist may be touching the cranium of the client, with the fingers cradling their occiput and the thumbs gently contacting the greater wings of their sphenoid. With the subtle and wholistic felt-sense of calm intensity, the therapist may start to perceive the subtle amplification of arising and passing at their own sphenoid bones, helping to open to the present moment unfolding of the client's wholistic tissue, fluid and potency expressions. In the same moment, the client will, at some level, feel this transmutation, although it is likely that they will interpret this as tissues shifting, or an ease of restriction, or 'energy' flowing within them or from the therapist.

> Q: Does this awareness of entanglement mean that we lose our midline sense of being an organism self and merge with the narrative of another?

Actually no, it is quite the reverse. This is because the therapist is perceiving change as the subtlest and most profound midline, as potency itself. This kind of perception is not merging into a narrative-based other. It is perceiving change as a relational unfolding in (of) the present moment.[8] So, when awareness acknowledges the patterns and rhythms of TI/ME, it is in effect perceiving the ingredients of experience as ephemeral,[9] whereas the identification of a narrative-based self is perceived as permanent. In other words, there is the insight that there is no permanent narrative to merge into or vice versa. Felt-sense insight in this regard is itself a midline preventing merging and therefore promoting health, i.e the awareness of change (potency).

This encourages the re-emergence of experienc*ing*[10] – presence free from assumptions based on TI/ME. At some point, this manner of relating will pervade with a wider perception, and open to a level of subtlety which is both dynamic and still, empty and full, nothing and everything, life and death. Wow – what a paradox! While the presence of calm intensity is touched by the insight of non-duality, this presence also touches the perspective of duality enough to realize the burden of delusion it carries with it. One needs to discover what one is, to discover what one is not.[11]

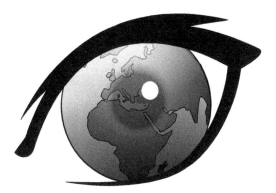

Figure 8.3: Insight in the 'act' of observation

8.4 Revelational realization

The most significant aspect of a treatment session often happens after the client has left the clinic and perhaps even when the therapist has returned home after the working day. Realizing this occurs concurrently with a huge shift in the therapist's understanding around the non-dual nature of dynamic stillness, and 'touching' this actuality is when the deepest changes unfold, both in the therapist and the client.

It can be hard to wrap one's head around this, and if one finally does then the thoughts, associating with various concepts, are nowhere near the reality of it. Still, the moment thought realizes its own limiting nature then potential understanding begins. So bearing this in mind, we will now inquire into it a little.

When the I/ME loop pattern (see Appendix 1) is perceived for what it is, it is the greatest opportunity a client's body can have to express health. This opportunity is amplified hugely when a therapist does not react to the I/ME loop. Such non-reaction will be at times easy and others hard. The reason for this is because the moment a therapist is aware of their own wholistic calm intensity expression, the I/ME loop will be severed, as TI/ME will be realized and understood as passing. But when a therapist feels a pattern in their own system, which is not obviously the client's pattern, then the therapist may be subconsciously reacting to the patterns in the client, which will consequentially disrupt the continuation of insight. Some consider this interruption 'somatic transference', which is a term that can distort the understanding of what is really taking place. It is quintessentially the therapist reacting to the client's patterns of experience because they believe they are their own patterns of experience.

Once a therapist understands this (after the client has left the clinic, or when they have returned home at the end of the working day), the tension, ache, heaviness, emotional charge, blurred vision, headache and so on can be 're-accessed' and witnessed with stillness. Sitting, lying or standing are all positions that can help, as long as one observes without intentional or reactive movement. This then invites the depth of stillness needed to reveal and nurture the reactive tendency, and for it to settle and encourage calm intensity to return, whereby dynamic stillness will be touched. Touch, in this manner, is deeply resourcing for the therapist and the client – actually it is resource itself.

Such after-work practice will help to dissipate the therapist's reaction and deepen their insight. Of equal importance, however, is the realization that this also settles the client's reactions, no matter where they are in the universe.[12]

Proximity-based bodywork produces felt-sense entanglement, whether our mind acknowledges it or not. It is then our responsibility, as a therapist, to follow through accordingly, depending on reactions we perceive in our own body. It could be considered nonchalant or even irresponsible to get home at the end of the day and distract oneself from the need to be still for some time. I am one of those who sees it like this as I have spent many years investigating the effects displayed by the client and myself, when I dedicate a period of time to being still at the end of the day – and when I don't. Over this period, it has become incredibly clear that an after-work stillness 'practice' is highly beneficial for the client, and also for one's own insight and deepening understanding of life. In this way, all clients can be seen as unknowingly helping a therapist deepen into insight.

So rather than seeing a client as a burden, or merely a means of earning income and putting bread on the table, such perspective nips suppressed countertransference tension in the bud. Furthermore, such practice also helps non-doing to be ever more embodied by the therapist and it becomes an automatic inclusion during a treatment session.

It will also become easier to notice inertial fulcrum patterns in the client during treatment sessions, as the therapist will be more and more familiar with their own reactive tendencies.

Another major benefit acquired by the therapist embodying stillness, in an environment with no distractions and solely with their own familiar presence, is the resource it provides to themselves during the working day. Many therapists reading this chapter might think this last statement is pretty obvious. However, it is surprising how few bodywork therapists set aside a period to let the deeper sensations bubble into the awareness of TI/ME passing. If sensations are identified with they will most often turn into reactive tendencies and these will then likely get buried as subconscious patterns in the body tissues and fluids. When this process continues, without perceiving sensations as they really are (arising and passing), it will consolidate as yet more TI/ME-based identification. This is a cycle which is hard to realize and one which many therapists and teachers furtively avoid or simply know nothing about.

Evidence of the lack of therapist self-care, in this regard, is provided here by the humble, yet well-known physician, Dr Gabor Maté[13]: a number of years prior to disclosing the following account Dr Maté had organized a health retreat, based on helping students to become familiar with ancient Peruvian traditional practices, in Peru. He flew down and met the traditional healers, whom he had not met before. Dr Maté was informed by the healers that he and his assistants were not in a fit state to help other people attending the retreat as their psycho-emotional physical states were too imbalanced, and they were likely to disrupt any deep health expression in those participating. It eventuated that Dr Maté and his assistants were first treated by the traditional healers to help the team establish a suitable body-mind balance before they continued with the retreat. Dr Maté is freely open in disclosing this event as he was impacted by realizing how normal an imbalanced system felt.

As health practitioners, we can benefit from this story by appreciating the importance of setting aside sufficient time (clock time), and finding a suitable environment, to realize TI/ME passing, even if we feel that our body-mind is already balanced.

Q: At what point do we invite the embodiment of non-doing into a session?

To answer this, we need to discover how and where TI/ME affects our sessions in order to notice where the perception of change is most needed. In other words, if we are reactively unengaged, TI/ME will flourish. Whereas if we regularly 'access' (engage with) our original nature, then the passing of TI/ME will be realized and non-doing will take over.

Try the following experiential exercise to evoke the understanding of when END is necessary.

◈ EXPERIENTIAL EXERCISE 12

Sensation dissolution
Laya dhyana

◆ In pairs: one person lies supine on the table aware of dissolution; one person acts as TI/ME, standing at the foot end of the table.

◆ Person on the table notices the dissolution of sensations with closed eyes.

◆ Person acting as TI/ME gently blows on any exposed skin on the body for five to ten seconds and repeats this anywhere without preparing the client, five to seven times on different areas of the body.

◆ Person on the table: is there a capacity to sense the dissolution of the sensation felt on the skin, before, during and after the blowing?

◆ Now the person acting as TI/ME gently touches an area of either the legs, abdomen, arms, head or face. Touch for five to ten seconds and repeat in five to seven different areas.

◆ Person on the table: can you sense the dissolution before, during and after the touch?

◆ Person acting as TI/ME gently tugs an aspect of the client's clothing in a manner which can be felt by the client for five to ten seconds.

◆ Person on the table: is dissolution present, before, during and after the tug?

◆ When you have finished, let the client lie with the sense of potential dissolution for a couple minutes, then swap around.

8.5 Seeing patterns with embodied non-doing

Seeing patterns with embodied non-doing (SPEND[14]) is not a technique and therefore not brought about by intent. Rather, it is the awareness a therapist has when there is sufficient insight of TI/ME passing. The more insight there is in the therapist, the more the client's patterns of experience will reveal themselves. A significant amplification of therapist insight occurs when the client's patterns can be perceived in their (the therapist's) body. This is a crucial aspect of the session for the therapist to appreciate as insight helps to increase the awareness of felt-sense entanglement. In a way, the therapist unintentionally 'exchanges' insight (calm intensity vibration of TI/ME passing) for the client's patterns which are ready to be shared. The deepest and most transmutational part of the session takes place in these moments. The vibration of insight, in the therapist, actually coaxes the sense of change in the client's system, rather than swapping or merging with anything. This can often feel like 'energy' coming from the therapist, so it is important for the therapist to remain present with the understanding of what is really happening so a client's misunderstanding can be reframed after the session, if needed.

Just as importantly, with this understanding and insight, the therapist can achieve what the client was unable to – that is to understand that the patterns are TI/ME and insightfully acknowledge the nature of TI/ME passing. So, in other words, the awareness of felt-sense entanglement is promoted by the therapist's insight of TI/ME passing, which is in effect both awareness and equanimity, and by not reacting to the patterns perceived, the tendencies of the client receive no support. With no support of reactive tendencies, the sensations are perceived as changing (perhaps energy by the client) – arising and passing.

The following metaphor may help to elucidate the last paragraph. If St George does not draw his sword, or run from the illusion of a dragon, then the dragon no longer draws support from St George to justify its existence. As the dragon disappears (passes) it stops blocking the nurturing vitality of the horizon – the potency of space is revealed and the insight of TI/ME passing is imbibed.

8.6 Five factors to help SPEND TI/ME

Factor one: Incorporating a visual, auditory or touch-based access point is very useful to establish stability for the mind. This can be a spot you see on the wall or a space you notice in the pattern on the carpet. It's good to keep the eyes open, if only a little bit, to avoid any tendency one might have to dissociate. The touch-based access point has already been mentioned (SASA).[15]

Factor two: Noticing the wide perceptual field, which may also be noticed as a long, slow rhythmic flow of potency. It is already present, so no need to intentionally expand awareness. Awareness is already expanded, but TI/ME funnels it into the impression of a separate self.

Factor three: Calm intensity, which, as mentioned, is the wholistic felt-sense of TI/ME passing.

Factor four: Felt-sense appreciation of client, which will require the establishing of the prior three factors.

Factor five: Equanimity, which, when truly integrated, will be realized as the essence of the other four factors. It is important here to appreciate what equanimity really means. Equanimity is not reacting to any sensation, be it pleasant or unpleasant, and noticing the passing nature of the sensation/s as a vibration/s which can be reciprocally felt by another. Established equanimity, therefore, helps the therapist reside in an interface of sensitivity to perceive the patterns of experience the client is subconsciously reacting to.

8.7 Elemental insight

For those who are new to the world of bodywork and resonate with a more elemental approach to perceived patterns, and the felt-sense of TI/ME passing, appreciating the following seven qualities may help. Also, if you are an experienced bodywork therapist and have become familiar with accessing the 'elements' (phases) via certain locations on or in the body (you may wish to call them ductless glands or *chakras*), then the felt-sense understanding of the following may be useful to better understand TI/ME passing:

1. Earth element (*muladhara*): Ground yourself. One simple way of establishing this is by sensing the earth with your feet (barefoot is always best), sitting with bones contacting the chair or floor. Earthing mats can be useful,[16] especially if in high-rise buildings or those which are very insulated from the earth. Another way is coming to a sense of the outline of your body. The felt-sense of the outline of your skin is a good way of appreciating this. There are many more but these two are useful as a foundation.

2. Water element (*swadhisthana*): Establish a felt-sense of the fluids in your body. This is a very useful way of coming to a sense of the whole and noticing that you are more than just the impression of your body outline.

3. Fire element (*manipura*): When you become aware of the continual transformation taking place at all levels, gross to extremely subtle, then the word transmutation will make sense. The gross is inherent with the potential expression of the subtle. The subtler a sensation is felt the more the transmutational quality is expressed. This is actually the transmutation of TI/ME by yielding to its nature, which is passing. Passing is potency and the potential of fresh and creative arising.

4. Air element (*anahata*): The balancing nature of the natural breath can be perceived both external and internal to the body, from the calm rising and lowering of the abdomen and chest to the subtle interchange of oxygen and carbon dioxide within the tissues and blood. Homeostasis presides just by being aware of this, and such awareness promotes balance, space and potency. This is a useful phase to 'reside' with when one has a propensity to sense subtle sound (*nada*).

5. Ether element (*vishuddhi*): Space, when perceived with the insight gleaned from the awareness of the prior two elements, will be empty of TI/ME rather than conceptual emptiness. It will be the realization of space being potency, a very valuable insight.

6. Insight (*ajna*): The insight of TI/ME passing is an inherent aspect of points 3, 4 and 5. When fire, air and ether elements are

established then insight of TI/ME passing in earth and water elements will be noticed also.

7. Wholeness (*sahasrara*): Now the insight of wholeness will be present – not just wholeness within one's own body but the wholeness provided by realizing the observer as the observed. This is a relational insight which enables the felt-sense of TI/ME passing in another person. All elements will now be perceived as expressive phases, but not separate.

It is good not to conceptualize, 'spiritualize' or romanticize these qualities of subtle expression too much. Otherwise, the insight of TI/ME passing will be overshadowed by the 'grey zone', in which case insight will be more difficult to 'develop' than if you were to start from scratch!

Chapter 9

Equanimity and the Grey Zone

*Our anxiety does not come from thinking about
the future, but from trying to control it.*

KHALIL GIBRAN

9.1 The importance of equanimity

The importance of understanding equanimity in therapeutic bodywork cannot be over-emphasized. Equanimity is of equal importance to awareness. Without awareness, we are blind to the world. Yet, without equanimity we have no capacity to investigate the depth of our being, as we will be continuously reacting to superficial stimulation and identifying ourselves with this superficiality.

When we sit still in a particular position for a period of time it is often quite nice to relax and let awareness reclaim its place in the present moment. However, after a while the undercurrent of the manifold patterns of experience start to surface. Awareness, by nature, cannot ignore what is arising and it is at this point that our tendency to do something comes into being. We either fidget, to alleviate a discomforting sensation, or we distract ourselves from a memory or experience by validating an excuse to get up and attend to a task of some sort, such as read a book, cook dinner, go to bed.

It is unfortunate that we rarely welcome the opportunity to practise our ability of not reacting to these arising sensations. If we were to explore the state of being aware, steady and still (*sthairyam*) we would notice that not only does our equanimity (*upekkha*) increase, but our awareness increases as well. With perseverance, the unsettling sensations become more tolerable and start to promote a sense of greater sensitivity, agency, depth and wholeness.

9.2 Distraction

Once a practitioner realizes that a subconscious reaction (to a sensation on or in the body) is a catalyst preventing deeper awareness, then the therapist also realizes that discriminating discernment (*viveka*) is necessary.

For example, during treatment, a question might arise in the practitioner's mind such as, 'Am I being a masochist by sitting through this pain in my back considering I sustained a disc prolapse a week ago?' Obviously, this is a situation which requires that the sensations of discomfort are listened and responded to appropriately.

Nevertheless, while messages highlighting danger are important to acknowledge, and respond to if necessary, they are rarely anything other than the mind reacting to a distractive tendency. In other words, most messages we receive from the mind, asking us to 'do' something, are prompts to distract us from what is surfacing from the depths of our subconscious.

> Q: So why does the mind do this?

The mind, through habit, will try to prevent deep TI/ME (Pli: *sankharas*; Skt: *samskaras*) from arising while attempting to perpetuate the familiar, superficial, known TI/ME, that is, the sensations we identify with and react on. Still, there is a deeper escape habit lurking. If the excuses are exhausted, and equanimity is weak, then the mind will often fall back on another option – it will dissociate![1] Dissociation, in such circumstances, is also a habit-prompting distraction, so it is also primed by intention.[2]

9.3 Tides of tantalization

Practitioner dissociation can become the most problematic feature in any sensation-based inquiry. This is because it can involve the tantalization of pleasure. Again and again, this feature enters into meditation practice around the globe. When it does, it is often considered to be meditation itself – it is not![3] At least not as far as this book's semantic understanding of the word meditation is concerned – meditation being the optimization of awareness, equanimity and resulting insight.

It is useful for a therapist to realize how this pleasure-seeking habit can enter our practice in the clinic room as it is an aspect of the grey zone which can obliterate equanimity and insight. When we are obligated to remain still during a treatment session, any excessive fidgeting will overtly void our credibility as an END practitioner. We therefore remain relatively still and aware of the unfolding sensations/expressions in both ourselves and the client. Discomfort may start to arise in our buttock cheeks, elbows and back, but we remain aware of the subtle nature of arising and passing as an undercurrent sensation. Don't we?

If we do not then it is likely, at some point during a treatment session, that we will (to some degree) dissociate from the sensations/expressions. Such dissociation can in fact feel relatively pleasant. The pleasant nature, in this case, is a dissociation-based reaction to avoid feeling reactive tendencies which have arisen during the session. It is at this point a therapist can enter the 'grey zone'.

In this situation, the mind needs to move, because mind *is* movement. It doesn't want to acknowledge the unfolding scene, so it (the mind) moves in a manner which befits the stimulation needed to catalyse a pleasant sensation, for example a subtle mind movement which promotes a physiologic opioid release. The client's system may resonate with the therapist's dissociation response and superficial calmness, but does this 'therapeutic state' help to calm down any underlying agitation in ourselves (which impacts the client)? No, the undercurrent of TI/ME will remain the same. Once pleasant calmness is felt by an individual, their system does not want or wish to return to the agitated state. Yet it will return, at some point, because the agitation is still there. In other words, the reprieve from agitated sensations, due to a pleasant sensation of being dissociated, has not provided any felt-sense insight into the nature of TI/ME passing.

If we are sane we will all prefer to have pleasure rather than pain. But this is exactly the point. Our tendency to prefer one sensation over another keeps us caught in a repetitive cycle – and results in a decreased threshold to tolerate unpleasant sensation.

Let's remember that we are here talking about ourselves as the practitioner. If we are not present to the reality of our own unfolding sensations then a client's system will start leaning towards dissociation as well; or the client will feel as if they are not being met.

The following ethological analogy is mentioned to help with understanding the relevance of an extremely subtle intent to dissociate. This is a survival strategy which is very relevant at the right time and the right place, but it is not a useful strategy to unconsciously blend into treatment sessions, or meditation sessions for that matter.

It is likely that a mouse will never fully go into a state of dissociation without the environment presenting imminent life-threatening danger (e.g. the close proximity of a fang-bearing cat, without possible escape). This is because dissociation is not good for its system. A mouse, for example, does not indulge in the pleasant sensations which nature provides to coerce it into staying still, and, if caught, does not flinch despite canine teeth biting through its flesh. Actually, any animal will eventually die if such dissociation is repeated often enough.

A practitioner who feels embodied and whole with the insight of arising and passing, in their own body, encourages the system of any client to feel safe enough to also explore their expressions – safe like an adapting river, not like a vault. This kind of perceived safety promotes potency expression rather than escaping experience by dissociating to preferred 'place'.

Conversely, if we demonstrate and declare the need for escape in our own system, a client's system will not feel confident to express its health. Establishing equanimity towards the pleasant sensations is much harder than equanimity towards the unpleasant sensations. It is, therefore, hugely beneficial to develop non-reactivity towards pleasant sensations whenever the opportunity arises.

So, TI/ME helps to provide limits and support consciousness as the individual organism orientates to the world of seeming things.

Of course, this relative world of duality will have its ups and downs, and the ups will lead to the downs. If these ups are translated into the therapeutic grey zone then this translation will become the obstacle to insight.

Now, having said all that, this does not mean that we should turn our backs on the day-to-day celebration of life. Pleasure is not the problem, it is the identification to the object which evokes the sensation that becomes the problem. For example, if we identify ourselves as a body (object) which is permanent and separate from other apparent objects, then the apparent pleasure we perceive will eventually become dissatisfactory, as the body is not permanent or essentially separate. However, when there is no identification, and only perception, then life unfolds as an incomparable adventure, always new, consciousness celebrating itself – first by forgetting 'itself' and then remembering 'itself' again in moments of profound clarity (insight). These are enlightened moments – truly conscious moments.

I remember a Zen teacher sharing how he couldn't imagine a more agonizing way to realize the nature of TI/ME passing[4] than to indulge in pleasure. It seemed so bizarre to him that anyone would adopt this approach to life over inquiring into the nature of being. He explained that in the 'act' of realizing TI/ME's inherent nature, of arising and passing, a joy far more meaningful than pleasure unfolds.

◆ EXPERIENTIAL EXERCISE 13

Taste equanimity
Upekkha rasa

◆ Place a succulent sweet on the middle of your tongue.

◆ Raise the tongue to the roof of your hard palate.

◆ Notice the taste of the sweet but don't swallow.

◆ Feel the sensations arising and passing in various areas of the body.

◆ Let the saliva build inside your mouth but don't swallow.

◆ Bring your awareness to the hyoid bone (floating bone beneath chin).

◆ Notice the space (akasha) here.

◆ Let this space, and the sensations arising due to not reacting, permeate the body and the space around you.

◆ Continue with this for another five minutes.

◆ Swallow the sweet – with equanimity.

◆ See how far you can sense the sweet descend down the oesophagus.

◆ What do you sense as an afterglow in your mouth?

◆ Do you get a sense of anything different regarding the sensations of your body?

◆ Is this different to the usual sense after swallowing something pleasant?

Figure 9.1: The taste of tantalization

CLINICAL NOTE

The perception of a pleasant sensation is one we are hardwired to want more of. Society tends to advertise the benefits of acquiring a sensation which feels pleasant. Hence, it is an automatic knock-on effect when we surreptitiously bring this desire for pleasant sensations into our clinical practice.

It is, therefore, very difficult to notice the arising and passing characteristic of pleasant sensations. Nevertheless, it is possible. Moreover, the awareness, equanimity and insight of these particular sensations enable the expression of calm intensity to develop and open to dynamic stillness.

9.4 Good/bad 'energy' trap

A therapist who reacts to sensations, by relishing the pleasant or building aversion to the unpleasant, or dissociating from the overwhelming, will eventually become trapped by the perception of individual clients having good or bad 'energy'. If a therapist embraces this dualistic perception they will in effect be 'gilding the lily'[5] or 'painting horns on the toad'[6] of potency. Potency is neither good or bad – it *is*.

We can live ordered and practical lives by perceiving the dualistic nature of objects in our environment. Yet, when we attempt to transfer this dualistic understanding to interpret the felt-sense of potency, then we bypass its essential reality and, therefore, miss the insight it has to offer. This will result in a therapist setting up an unbalanced relational field in the clinical setting, and prevent sessions from unfolding with their optimal potential. Moreover, this dualistic reactivity will increase the likelihood of psychological transference and countertransference issues entering therapy sessions. Such perspective will leave a therapist feeling elated after one session and drained after another, which will provide limited work-life motivation and longevity for the clinician.

9.5 Potency awareness versus energy manipulation

Another grey area that can present itself is when a therapist perceives potency but thinks that they have control over it. Controlling potency is merely the mind setting up an image, based on the felt-sense, and then distorting the image in time and perceived space. This is what we are doing all the time with objects and experiences, usually to good effect, as we can manipulate what we know in our minds and plan our day according to our practical needs and preferences. But, potency is not an experience – it is experienc*ing*. In other words, one cannot remember potency. As soon as one tries to it is not potency, it is TI/ME.

Therefore, if a therapist's intention is involved with moving potency, then they are not practising with equanimity or from insight.

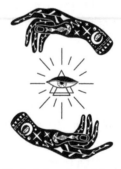

Figure 9.2: Esoteric hands and droopy third eye

9.6 Insight, the distinction between calm intensity and dissociation

The antidote to becoming mesmerized by grey-zone intention is insight – insight of the nature of nature (insight of the nature of potency).

In other words, the insight of arising and passing and the subsequent dissolution of TI/ME.

The insight of arising and passing eventually results in the complete dissolution of TI/ME. Such awareness, equanimity and insight is calm intensity (not dynamic stillness) which interfaces with the non-dual absoluteness of dynamic stillness. Calm intensity is receptive and non-reactive in the 'realm' of TI/ME (relative reality) as well as non-duality (absolute reality). It is important to note that the insight of TI/ME passing is not dissociation from TI/ME. Dissociation is a physiologic survival strategy, which can become a psychologic tendency if repeated enough, and is a big trap which many 'meditators' get caught by. Yogis who are well versed in the affects of dissociation know that dissociating from TI/ME can be helpful for attaining a deeply relaxed state. Nevertheless, these yogis also realize that they need to re-embody themselves, at which time they discover that TI/ME is exactly as it was before they entered the trance (dissociated). Therefore, there has been no insight. The methods some yogis use to re-establish embodiment (awareness of physical sensations and TI/ME) can be austere, such as immersing in ice cold water, or adopting contorted physical postures. Yet, these austerities, if not balanced, can also become the catalyst for increasing the tendency to dissociate. So practices like this can become a problematic loop, encouraging more and more disembodiment/ dissociation, which means that dissociation becomes a surreptitious intention. In other words, it becomes a desire to escape from TI/ME rather than opening to the non-doing insight of TI/ME passing. The key qualities of distinction between dissociation and calm intensity are awareness of body sensations, arising and passing, and choice. The state of partial or full dissociation is absent of these qualities, whereas the 'state' of calm intensity is endowed with all of them.

In various dictionaries the term dis*ass*ociation is used instead of dissociation. It means the same thing, despite having one extra syllable. Nevertheless, perhaps a semantic difference between the two could help with understanding the (huge) difference between dissociation and calm intensity. Dis*ass*ociation from the awareness of sensation awareness, in this semantic perspective, has an opposite called re-association of sensation awareness. However, dissociation from the awareness of sensations has an opposite called calm intensity, which is the awareness of sensations and the insight of their nature being to arise and pass away. The opposite of dis*ass*ociation (re-association) would therefore reaffirm identity but compound the sense of permanence and separation. This is profoundly different from the opposite of dissociation (calm intensity), where there would be a sense of identity and felt-sense relationship with the insight of impermanence that is beyond the illusion of identification.

Siddhartha Gautama (Gotama), the historical Buddha, realized the dilemma of, on the one hand, common people orientating towards object-based self-gratification, and, on the other hand, the austere yogis orientating towards a state of self-mortification and dissociation. Consequently, he discovered (some would say rediscovered) what he termed 'the middle path' (*majjhima patipada*). To overcome these outlined extremes of perspective he recommended his followers practise a form of attentive awareness on the body (*kaya-nupassana*), body-mind sensations (*vedana-nupassana*), mind (*citta-nupassana*) and mental contents (*dhamma-nupassana*), and to be aware of their arising and passing nature (insight). He recommended that the majority of formative meditation be on the breath, or an object which helped to encourage a state of access attention (*upacara-samadhi*) which neighbours the state of being absorbed (dissociating). While they were in this neighbourhood conscious 'state', the gathering insight of impermanence would help the follower realize subtler and subtler phenomena arising and passing (Pli: *dhamma*; Skt: *dharma*).

Sometimes, yogis from other traditions would hear what the Buddha was teaching and travel from far and wide to become followers. Often, they would have tendencies to dissociate due to their past practices, especially the extremely ascetic yogis. This tendency was, in fact, sometimes a benefit rather than a hindrance as the methods of deep concentration they used to attain an absorbed state were occasionally a useful form of concentration to sustain neighbourhood consciousness for long periods of time, and, therefore, were able to glean the insight of very subtle phenomena arising and passing.

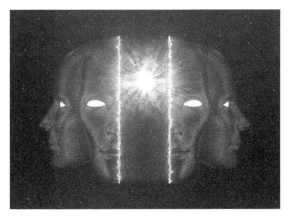

Figure 9.3: Insight, the distinction between calm intensity and dissociation

◆ EXPERIENTIAL EXERCISE 14

Heart space equanimity
Hridayakasha upekkha

◆ Bring your awareness to your chest.

◆ Open to the space in this region.

◆ Let the awareness of this space simultaneously acknowledge and accommodate the wider perceptual field.

◆ Notice the potency deep to the heart space.

◆ Is there a good or bad quality to the felt-sense of this potency? Be patient when answering this.

◆ Do you notice yourself wanting to do something with the potency you perceive? Do you want more or less? For it to be in another area or everywhere?

◆ When you notice the reactive tendencies of the mind then potency has a chance to show itself fully. It is like potency no longer needs to be shy.

◆ Chapter 10 ◆

Engaged Non-Doing

Nature does not hurry, yet everything is accomplished.

LAO TZU

10.1 END principles

Engaged/embodied non-doing (felt-sense connection) is the essence of body therapy. It is neither a *laissez faire* form of passive nonchalance or an escape of the mind to another realm of perception. Nor is it trying not to 'do', as this is also a form of 'doing'.

Well-trained biodynamic craniosacral therapists tend to have a fairly good understanding of non-doing. The word biodynamic is a good word to use to describe the non-doing felt-sense of the expression of health and the process of returning to our original nature.[1]

We have established that non-doing is the term used (in this context) to describe being aware and not reacting to sensation, TI/ME or its outcome, i.e. intention (see Appendix 1). Yet, to some, it may seem preposterous to promote a treatment which has no intention. To the devout hard materialist,[2,3] the idea of this could amount to mindlessness, whereas to the 'unique' new-age esotericist the idea could seem like failing to ask for special energy from the pleiades angels.[4] Yet, if we look at both viewpoints, it can be seen that it is the very nature of ideation which prevents the understanding of what non-doing really is.[5] Engaged non-doing is a presence which cannot be labelled or categorized, much to the frustration of a mind that abstractly conceptualizes consciousness as existing solely due to matter forming the mind.

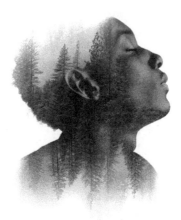

Figure 10.1: The effortless effort of nature presenting itself

Another way of understanding this can be by acknowledging the limits of the mind. The following Zen koan can help us to realize the limitations of intention and the profound simplicity of felt-sense non-doing free from ideation:

> If a person puts a baby goose (gosling) in a bottle and feeds it until it is full-grown, how can the goose be free without it being killed or breaking the bottle?

This is a conundrum/riddle that has been dished out to Zen monks for several hundred years. Koans are not supposed to be easy. They have been described as a practice to provoke 'the great doubt', and test a student's progress towards enlightenment. The rationale is to sit with an utterly illogical situation, gnawing away at it with the reasoning part of your mind, until finally the mind yields further attempts at analysis and makes a quantum leap into 'pure consciousness' (*purusha*). Most notably, Zen teachers do not expect their students to present a straight-forward answer to a koan. To illustrate, here is an example of the response a great Zen master (called Nansen) gave to his acolyte (called Riko) when presented with what is known as the 'goose koan':

After hearing the riddle, Nansen gave a huge clap with his hands and shouted, 'Riko!'

'Yes, master,' said the student with a shock.

'Ah…see,' said Nansen. 'The goose is out!'

This can seem like gibberish. What weirdo would put a gosling into a bottle to grow in the first place? How would it eat and breathe as it gets bigger? The mind is already getting too involved to answer the koan! And the mind of the student will generally escalate from there with all kinds of theories and conceptual gymnastics:

- The bottle lacks a tapered neck so the goose can get out whenever it needs to.

- The goose is fed so sparingly by its sadistic owner that its emaciated body is able to come and go as it pleases.

- A laser cutter could slice carefully through the glass without touching the goose, thus freeing it.

- The bottle can be melted in such a way that it doesn't harm the goose but ensures its freedom.

The student's mind can continue for years with one koan and deepen further and further into this conceptual frenzy. The real answer erupts when the pressure of the student's mind gives up on finding an answer and realizes the passing nature of TI/ME when this happens.

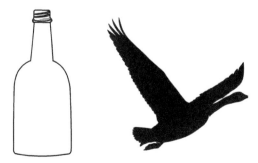

Figures 10.2a and 10.2b: Bottle and goose

From an END perspective, the goose symbolizes our consciousness, our source, our ultimate reality, while the bottle represents our mind formed by TI/ME. This koan suggests that consciousness is trapped inside the mental structures of our logical, analytical mind. If we want to experience the ultimate freedom of pure consciousness, liberation and dynamic stillness, we need to give up and release the process of asking rational questions and generating logical solutions. When we can relinquish and just 'be', without the mental narration, only then will 'the goose be free'.

So, the practitioner needs to be aware of the felt-sense of arising and passing, especially passing. TI/ME cannot exist in the felt-sense presence of embodied non-doing – the awareness of arising/passing – only experienc*ing* can.

10.2 Dissolution of TI/ME

'Blessed are the meek, for they will inherit the earth,' Matthew 5:5.

END version: 'Those in touch with the subtlest shall embody the expression of the universe.'

So, TI/ME dissolves into the felt-sense of passing and passing with insight and engenders fresh arising – arising and passing being our inherent reality, and TI/ME being its dualistic representation. TI/ME is obviously very useful as it helps us orientate to the environment as separate individuals. Yet, as has been mentioned, it dominates our perspective of the world when we identify with reactive tendencies associated to it.

Overriding tendencies, therefore, distort our perception and leave our inner being dissatisfied with what we are left with. It is a bit like a parched traveller spotting water in a desert, only to find when they reach the seeming origin of the mirage that there is nothing to quench their thirst. Similarly, an END practitioner will not meet a client with clarity if intention is the presiding factor underpinning the relational contact. This is because intention sustains TI/ME and obscures the felt-sense of arising and passing. However, do not fret if TI/ME persists without passing; if you are conscious of TI/ME's recalcitrance then you are already benefiting from half of what is needed to notice it passing. Equanimity is the other half and this will establish itself with patient perseverance.

It is truly invigorating when a client's body wakes up to the dissolution of TI/ME. This is encouraged and inspired by the practitioner's embodied awareness. Nevertheless, it is possible that a client may feel agitated with the initial sense of TI/ME passing, or they may occasionally be overwhelmed due to re-associating with the arising sensations which they originally suppressed. If this occurs when we are aligned and in touch with a felt-sense of calm intensity (in ourselves) then spontaneous verbal guidance often tends to present itself to help resource the client. Such verbal guidance is the insight of non-duality enabling a balanced verbal expression in duality. We may say something to help guide the client to find resource, or perhaps we remain silent. The relational intelligence somehow knows what needs to be said. In this circumstance, a key thing to understand is that insight is calling the shots, not intention.

Perhaps a client will come back the following session and say that they have been on a roller-coaster ride (metaphorically), which you and they did not suspect. Does this mean you have failed to pick up on something? Possibly, and yet also possibly not. If you are in touch with insight rather than intention, then nothing will have been missed.

When a client's system is waking up to suppressed sensations, and feeling the surfacing of held patterns of experience, then the client's dislike of the arising sensations needs to be explained, and perhaps managed, but not viewed and reinforced as a problem. This is important to understand, and it may be that a large part of the next session is spent focusing and resourcing techniques in order to help accommodate the unpleasant sensations. Eventually this should taper off to resume the essence of our practice and the real reason for the client attending sessions – re-connecting to health. But all the while the practitioner is in touch with the insight of calm intensity and the felt-sense of fluids within the fluids.[6]

The Pali word for the felt-sense insight of calm intensity is *sampajanna*. With correct meditation guidance and understanding the full body felt-sense of *sampajanna* can then open to a sense of full-body dissolution called *bhanga*. In Theravada Buddhist literature[7] the tangible meaning of this word is only discovered when one interprets one's own felt-sense with insight (nature of arising and passing), and investigates the changing nature of one's own body sensations with awareness and equanimity.

One verse from the *Visudhimagga*[8] goes as follows:

> He (the monk) reaches contemplation of dissolution by abandoning arising. When all formations have been realized, due to the contemplation of their incessant dissolution (passing), he becomes dispassionate towards them (drops intention), his greed for them fades away and he is liberated from them (realizes non-duality).

This may sound a little too religious for your reading palette. Still, it is useful to acknowledge what a verse like this means and that this understanding and insight has been circulating for at least 2500 years. Nonetheless, it seems likely that it has been distorted, misunderstood and ignored innumerable times.[9] Calm intensity is, therefore, not just theory (*pariyatti*), it is deep felt-sense insight (*patipatti*).

◆ EXPERIENTIAL EXERCISE 15

Passing at third ventricle
Laya ajna mudra

◆ Place the thumb tip of one hand at the philtrum.

◆ With fingers together raise the little finger two centimetres and focus the eyes on the nail.

◆ After three minutes, remove the hand and gaze at the impression formed in the mind.

◆ When the impression starts to dissolve, notice the process of dissolution.

◆ Are you aware of the dissolution?

◆ Once it has gone, notice the clarity of the empty space it leaves behind.

◆ Also notice the mind wanting to replace this space with something.

◆ Finally, notice the subtle body sensations resonating with the space.

10.3 The non-doing sage

During the twentieth century, an outstanding individual tirelessly alluded to the importance of calm intensity insight (for almost 60 years). His name was Jiddu Krishnamurti (1895–1986). He was an influential inspiration for many of the original biodynamic craniosacral therapy pioneers, including Rollin Becker.[10] He emphasized the point that thought contains a tendency to move away from its natural designation, and when it does it prevents insight. Krishnamurti recommended that thought should not attempt to get into the area of spiritual, love, beauty or even truth as it would be trying to *make* permanent an expression which is manifestly impermanent.

In addition to this, discussions he and the illustrious quantum theory scientist Professor David Bohm[11] had in the latter years of his life helped some people to understand his explanation of how the subtlety of thought envokes deep delusion when it takes control of the nervous system.

They established that this control of the nervous system probably originated when primitive humans began to have an increased capacity to think, and at this point wanted to find something more than its 'limits' (due to their dissatisfactory nature). In other words, thought wants to feel better, or more, but cannot perceive the self-deception which it uses to make this happen.

During some of his many talks Krishnamurti asked his audience the following question, put in different ways: 'Can an individual free themselves from all self-centredness and self-delusion and feel that beyond the limits of thought? If so, the nervous system may be able to change by itself.'

Professor Bohm, whenever present, would often remind Krishnamurti that a functional centre (thought) is needed to operate as an animate being, and Krishnamurti would agree. However, they both concurred that this centre needs to know its limits, and be comfortable with non-doing in order for insight to present itself (thought fuelled by insight). Yet, they continued, thought is often unwilling to acknowledge non-doing as an option, because it would concurrently need to accept uncertainty. So, intention and the acceptance of uncertainty cannot co-exist.

In other words, when thought tries to provide security (safe like a vault), in a 'dimension' which does not accommodate such safety, conflict occurs. This conflict prevents the felt insight of love, beauty, 'spirit', connectedness and truth from expressing itself. Krishnamurti, therefore, was emphasizing that the essence of connecting with oneself, and another, requires the insight of knowing the limits of TI/ME by sensing its ephemeral (passing) nature. In addition to this, he stressed that non-doing (not reacting) acts as a gateway for felt-sense connection to present itself.

He also noted the importance of distinguishing secure developmental attachment[12] from psychologic attachment in the post-adolescent years. This is imperative for the healthy development of the nervous system in the formative years of life[13] and to enhance the vitality of deep relationship. Yet, the subconscious human mind insidiously hijacks this physiologic need and uses it as a way to reinforce the TI/ME of psychologic identity.[14] This may establish a sense of safety, but this is the kind of safety akin to a vault, not a flowing river (again, remember we are here talking in the context of ourselves as therapists, whereas clients will often need to re-establish secure attachment in order for health to express itself).

It is as if the mind keeps trying to repeat the benefits of developmental attachment year on year by placing more and more dependence on an object, activity, person, substance and so on. Contemporary social psychologists call this 'motivated reasoning', whereby any facts which oppose the perceived benefits are resisted or ignored. Unfortunately, this cycle won't let us open to the deeper aspects of why the developmental attachment took place in the first place. Neurophysiologists and psychologists focus on the development of physiologic and mental health, but rarely do they consider the early attachment as being a catalyst helping to support the contact with our original nature, the essence of relationship.[15]

Each successive year, tendencies, leading to intention and attachment, support an identity based on accumulation and dependence rather than feeling the essence of humanness.[16] When this happens, the insight and intimacy of our original nature become less and less apparent. Put the other way around, if we connect with another person, activity, substance, object, with ever-decreasing attachment, then our original nature will increasingly show itself. Nevertheless, if we try to abandon attachment, it will itself become another pursuit leading to other forms of attachment.

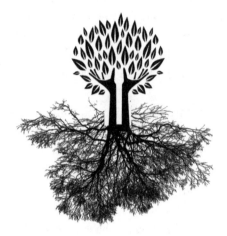

Figure 10.3: Non-centred wholeness and centre of expression

10.4 Insight-primed primal midline

To access the depth where self and no-self meet the felt-sense of the primal midline is key, especially during treatment sessions. When we are treating a client, the awareness of this midline will encourage a subtler level of body-based listening. Moreover, when we are aware of the primal midline with insight (TI/ME passing), the client's body gets a chance to be resourced at a much deeper level. This is because the client will not be receiving a reaction (from you) to their subconscious reactions.

This kind of listening will result, at some level, in the client listening to you listening. Thus you can now listen to them listening to you listening. What a great space for their body-based patterns to express themselves! We are not talking 'good or bad' here, we are talking about their patterns arising and you providing a neutral listening platform for the passing of their reactions to take place. This kind of relational listening is not engendering attachment or detachment, it is providing insight into the natural flow of the stream of health.

Whole-body dissolution (calm intensity) is your ultimate midline – it is the fluid/potency river itself. This is the connection base which encourages the client's inertial fulcra to release and for potency to reintegrate any fragmentation so that health can express itself.

It may be that the sense of arising and passing insight in your body starts to wane. When this happens, come to the sense of your primal midline. When you have been present with calm intensity, the orientation to the primal midline will establish a somatic representation of duality and, paradoxically, non-duality. This is the ultimate perceptual paradox, yet one that is entirely grounded.

In other words, the primal midline, perceived in you, with the insight of arising and passing, will enable fresh thought to arise at the same time. This differs to conventional thought and thinking, because it will now be fuelled by insight rather than TI/ME – what a thought!

The words which you speak, while in contact with such potency (insight of arising and passing), will always be appropriate and encouraging for the client's system to balance and reorganize.

◆ EXPERIENTIAL EXERCISE 16

Primal midline
Ashwini mudra

Sit comfortably. Kneeling is ideal, but not essential (if deciding to kneel use a cushion or pillow between the legs if it is uncomfortable).

◆ Notice the natural breath.

◆ Feel the unintentional touch of the breath, if possible.

◆ Start to gently contract and release your anal sphincter muscle.

◆ Hold for a second and release for a second.

◆ With rhythm, repeat this for a minute while practising bhuchari mudra.

◆ After a minute, contract one last time and hold it.

◆ Close the eyes and lower the hand while inhaling and hold the breath for seven seconds.

◆ Be aware of the third-eye impression or space (*bahir chidakasha*) and the upward expression of the primal midline.

◆ Exhale while releasing the sphincter muscle.

◆ Notice the natural inclination not to breathe back in. Don't force it, just be aware of the natural ease of not needing to breathe.

◆ What is the felt-sense of the body while not needing to breathe?

◆ Has the primal midline changed from being 'in' the body to being the whole itself?

10.5 Warrior *wu wei* versus wimpy wistlessness

It is a mistake to consider non-doing as inactive. Insight provides non-reactivity (non-doing) with an incredible 'empty of doing' vitality, and is not at all a form of passive dissociation. Understanding this difference is important, yet rare, due to our entrenched belief that a doing mind is a useful mind propelled by *a-priori* and *a-posteriori* reasoning. Yet, a reasoned thought with no verifying experience is merely temporal activity, void of felt-sense, and the resulting thoughts lead to conclusions which are merely mental activities caught in TI/ME.

It is important to understand this, as a client's system will know whether you are embodied and present or not, and sense either the presence of a nurturing warrior or a reactive mind propelled by agitation and lacklustre illusions.

10.6 Choice, insight and choicelessness

Choice is the act of choosing between two or more possibilities. We live in a society which not only encourages this act but also conveys the idea that our very well-being depends on it. Indeed, it would seem crazy to say that having no choice is a better situation to be in. Nevertheless, a fundamental aspect of choice requires there to be a preference for one possibility over the other(s). This means that there needs to be a relative psychologic base of what is liked and disliked, what is good, bad; right, wrong, and so on. Although the practical nature of these opposites gives direction to our lives, they also embolden the impression of our sense of being a seperate self. The sense of being a separate self fragments awareness and, consequently, prevents the sense of wholistic awareness. Wholistic awareness is by nature choiceless, and all the magic of nature expresses itself as such.

So, the practical relevance of choice promotes the impression of there being a chooser, which, relatively speaking, is a useful impression to have. However, the actuality of choiceless awareness is freedom from the world of choice and provides insight into the relative and absolute worlds. Insight, in this regard, is the interface awareness which touches both worlds. In a way, it is the 'realm' of the ultimate choice, i.e the choiceless choice of attending to the practicalities of choice or settling into the nature of dynamic stillness free from the delusion of a choice maker and empty of self-fed intention.

10.7 Subatomic and molecular touch

Empty touch is the touch of non-doing. The mind which is empty of self-fed intention promotes the insight of TI/ME passing, i.e. the awareness of awareness. This does not mean that the body's chemical reactions cease, actually it is the reverse. In the moment of realizing that there is not a permanent seperate self, molecular expression is enhanced and awareness is freed from the shackles and illusion of TI/ME. When molecular interactions are free from TI/ME, the felt-sense of oneself (organism-based self) and another is, in effect, the unique expression of one whole system communicating with itself.

Despite the potential awareness of this wholeness, there can be inhibiting factors which are dependent on the medium by which we are extrinsically communicating. For example, while interacting with another, via a medium such as the internet, the visual and auditory senses would feed information to the mind and the mind would do all the things a mind 'does' to continue the interaction. If an individual were to be aware of their own bodily sensations as the meeting progressed it may become apparent that the body begins to get confused at the molecular level. This is because there is a lot of particular information entering these dominant senses, but contradictory information entering the molecular validation sense organs (MVSOs). These MVSOs include the sense of smell, and pheromonal verification units such as the vomeronasal organ, for those who have one which is operational. During a visual/verbal online chat, the sense of smell is receiving information which conflicts with the information received by the eyes and ears. Another sense which receives information, ambivalent to what is seen and heard, is the exquisitely subtle sense of touch, which is usually acquired via felt-sense proximity to another. This forms a perfect storm for TI/ME to step in and fragment the internal molecular awareness of the body.

It might be useful to consider the following: while the sense of smell[17] and touch are interested in any molecular change in the proximity-based environment, the visual and auditory senses are sensitive enough to receive and relay the even subtler information of photons and phonons. It is the conditioned mind which translates this into something understandable and, therefore, potentially practical. Yet, as mentioned, such perception, without non-contradictory MVSOs, will result in TI/ME becoming more entrenched.

The last paragraph implies that as a race we generally perceive 'things', which results in substantiating the perspective of a permanent and separate self. Although this is a practical perspective it also obscures insight. In other words, we substitute the wholeness of non-duality with the fragmentation of duality and ignore the insight of calm intensity.

EXPLORATORY QUESTIONS FOR THE END THERAPIST

What would happen, during certain proximity-based interactions, if the visual and auditory senses acted as a perceptual gate to enhance photon and phonon 'information' without the influence of TI/ME?

What if the molecularly sensitive senses were predominantly meant to interpret grosser dualistic interactions while the subtler senses predominantly provide the mirror-like vibration for the insight of the non-dual 'world'?

An interesting point here is that the sense of interoception seems to be molecularly sensitive and primed for survival, while also being 'subatomically' sensitive enough to perceive responses deeper than those needed for survival, and appreciate wholeness. The insight of being present with the latter kind of touch provides the therapist with a felt-sense of calm intensity, which is the interface of choice and choicelessness.

For those who are struggling with trying to understand this, I recommend letting the conceptual mind be occupied by reading or listening to a relevant book/audio book.[18] While this is by no means a substitute for the intimate understanding gleaned by the experiential exercises outlined in this book, it can act as a palatable review to help calm the conceptual mind with an appropriate theme, perhaps appropriate enough to let thought realize its own limits. If so, you're back on board.

The following four chambers of non-doing may help simplify what has been read until this point and translate it into a form of clinical orientation. It is to be hoped that this simplification can be understood without dumbing down the profundity of it, because ultimately it is the insightful felt-sense vitality of 'This' which is far more simple than conceptual simplicity.

10.8 Four chambers of non-doing orientation

The following 'chambers' have already been covered in the guise of calm in-10-city and five factors of insight. But the following may help simplify a therapist's orientation during clinical practice.

Chamber 1: The access/balance point

If it feels that there is too much doing taking place with the access point of choice then rest your eyes on a small but definable object or impression in the room in which you are treating. If you observe this for some time the mind will generally become less 'doey' and balanced. I like to put a few strategically placed sticky black dots on the white wall of my clinic in case I need a simple external reference. I also find that it becomes easy to be aware of this and the natural breath on the philtrum at the same time. A point of caution should be noted here: if you have a tendency to get 'absorbed' by visual objects and mental images then it is better to remain with the natural sensations evoked by stimulus on the body as an access/balance point.

Chamber 2: Insight field

As mentioned, preparatory access point awareness will begin to open to the subtle sense of arising and passing on and in the body. While this is becoming more appreciable, the wider perceptual field will start to unveil itself naturally. During a treatment session, if you feel that more space would be useful for the client to deepen and they are feeling resourced, then become aware of your auditory sense and open to 'white noise' and 'vibrant silence'. The wide perceptual field is there.

Chamber 3: Calm intensity

This chamber is the amalgamation of three to seven if compared to the ten points of 'calm in-10-city'. If calm intensity is present then felt-sense connection, change and health will follow.

Chamber 4: END

When there is a felt-sense connection, the body comes back into contact with its intelligence. It will seem as though you can feel the client's sensations as separate from you and at times as not separate from you and at other times as both separate and not separate from you.

If you remain aware of calm intensity then you are also with your midline (they are the same). END *is* felt-sense connection.

NB: All four chambers have potential to include the fifth insight factor, equanimity. This chamber presents an eternal freedom to all metaphoric chambers, stages, levels, categories and so on, whatever they may be.

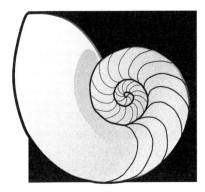

Figure 10.4: The chambers with no limits

10.9 Felt-sense connection

There can be a potential misinterpretation of what is here being called 'felt-sense connection'. If the first three chambers of non-doing are not established then there is a possibility that the perceived 'somatic resonance' (felt-sense connection) is in fact a form of therapist-induced 'somatic countertransference'. This is established subconsciously by the therapist as an attempt to justify patterns of experience arising from within their own system, either during conversation or while silently treating, due to triggered memories and/or emotions presenting themselves in the mind. For this reason, it is hugely beneficial to become familiar with one's own patterns so when they arise they are not projected as being the client's patterns. That way the therapist will be intimately aware of the passing nature of TI/ME, and the client's body will feel met (listened to) as the real attuned felt-sense connection establishes itself.

A good example of how attuning to the felt sense in oneself provides somatic resonance with another is provided by the following true account.

An event took place at a mental health ward in the Hawaii State Hospital, whereby all the patients were said to be cured by one man called Dr Ihaleakala Hew Len. The most amazing part is that he didn't see a single patient.

Reportedly, the patients were totally out of control and the ward where the patients were kept was known to be a very dangerous place. Some psychologists would leave on a regular basis and the staff would often call in with excuses not to come to work. People tentatively did their rounds full of fear of the prospect of being attacked by the patients. It was an unsafe environment which provided little inspiration to those working there.

Primarily, Dr Len was asked if he could help with the instability of the ward because of his reputation of being well versed in an ancient spiritual technique called *ho'oponopono*. It was more of a courtesy call at first, but when changes in the ward manifested people started to take Dr Len seriously.

He agreed to see what he could do and subsequently worked there for three years. By the end of that time the ward was closed because all the patients had healed!

Dr Len didn't see any of the patients professionally, nor did he counsel them. He only arranged to review and study their files. While he perused their files, he would establish the issues of the patients in himself and notice the effect that loving equanimity had rather than analysis or judgement. He would also repeat a mantra, of sorts, many times, asking to be freed from any karmic separation to the essence of the client. In other words, he was asking to be freed from any reactive tendencies he had which prevented him from feeling connection to the client. Miraculously, the entire ward began to 'heal'.

After a few months of Dr Len being there, patients who had been heavily medicated started getting their medications reduced. Those who had been chained were given permission to walk freely; and, most notably, those patients who had been labelled as being unreleasable were being freed. Furthermore, the staff stopped avoiding work. The ward ended up having more staff than were needed and skipping off work became very rare, mostly because patients were being released.[19]

Dr Len was asked what the *ho'oponopono* approach was in essence. His reply was: 'Love.'

Rewording Dr Len's understanding of the context of embodied non-doing therapy we might see that when the passing of TI/ME is realized as the expression of health, this very realization is also the deepest connection we have to our own, and another's, essence. The essence is: 'This' (the insight of TI/ME arising and passing).

If someone alludes to talking about 'This' by describing the differing traits they see or feel in another, then they are not talking about 'This'. Moreover, if somebody reacts to someone else's potency, for example by physically taking a step back due to the powerful energy of another, then they are not with the insightful (non-reactive) contact of 'This'.

There is a Taoist word *tzu jan* (*ziran*) which means the insightful intimacy that comes about when nature is 'permitted' to exist and develop without interference or conflict. *Tzu jan* is 'This'.[20] 'This' is the love which has no opposite.

There are some who propose *tzu jan* is the 'I AM' feeling. This interpretation may be accurate, when insight is deeply intertwined with the words which are being shared. However, it can often be misleading for people hearing this, especially when the listener, or reader, is not in felt-sense proximity to the person sharing the words. If the term 'I AM' becomes a projection of TI/ME then all kinds of egoic mischief can be justified by the mind. One then becomes content residing in a metaphoric prison cell, decorating the windows and walls with the projection of wholeness, rather than realizing its vibrant reality. However, there are, and have been, non-dual teachers who are quite remarkable in their ability to impart the *vedantic/tantric* understanding of 'I AM' which then becomes a deeply enriching application of daily life experiencing and insight. Conversely, there are those who interpret 'No I' as a belief, rather than felt-sense insight, and can dwell in a semi-dissociated torpor, hesitant to engage socially; whereas 'No I' is an extremely deep and insightful revelation which inspires a sharing with the 'heart' of society.

CLINICAL NOTE

I find felt-sense connection to be particularly demonstrable when babies and parents attend my clinic. More often than not it is the mother who brings her baby and remains in the room while the baby is being treated. If the baby is settled enough for the mother to relax, and observe the treatment at a distance, then a display of overt felt-sense connection commonly presents itself. This happens when the baby enters a calm 'state' which subsequently reminds the mother of her own calmness. The mother then starts to doze into a state of being half awake, half asleep, while the baby's body then begins to subtly shift and re-organize. When the shifts are particularly overt, I often witness the mother mirror the same slight movements, despite the fact that her eyes are closed and her being seemingly asleep.

It is my view that this subtle mirroring is about the point where the neurophysiological mirror neurone mimicry tapers into something much more subtle and fluid-like.

When one truly understands the observer as the observed,[21] whether it be a seeming animate or inanimate object, then the term 'This Is' cannot be interpreted in any other way than as a reminder to the calm yet vibrant felt-sense of wholeness.

So, some people seem to interpret the felt-sense of 'I AM' as equating, essentially, to realizing our essence is 'This' (in the context outlined in this book). Similarly, there are those who appear to express understanding of the felt-sense of 'No I' as equating, essentially, to 'This Is'. Therefore, the phrase 'This Is' may help unify the understanding of these seemingly different perspectives into a perspective which is essentially the same – the insight of TI/ME passing to reveal our original nature and connectedness to all beings (actually even non-beings).

10.10 This Is[22,23]

Insight is neither this nor that – yet, This Is insight.

This is very very near – closer than that, it is actually here.

This cannot be fragmented or fractured, yet This is the essence of TI/ME.

There is no beginning or end to This, yet This is the beginning of everything, including TI/ME.

This has no structure, but all structures are founded on This.

This is eternal, yet mortal in the formed perception of TI/ME.

This-ness is knowing.

This is in everything we do and don't do, but it is only in non-doing we realize This.

This *is* love and loves all that exists, yet its essence is not limited by existence.

In seeing, This sees.

In hearing, This hears.

In smelling, This smells.

In tasting, This tastes.

In touching, This touches.

In knowing, This knows.

This is This in all apparent things, while eternally whole and infinitely complete.

The arising perception of an object is the appreciation of This expression itself, and its passing nature reflecting the reality of This...as This.

A mirage of limitations, in an ocean of potential.

This-ness is beaming :)

This cannot be objectified – yet realizing the passing nature of objects is the insight of This.

This cannot be perceived – yet we perceive This alone.

We could invest a lifetime trying to understand This, yet This cannot be understood.

This is full, but is empty – has nothing, but contains all there is.

This offers everything – but is never drained or depleted.

This is a division-less movement, which heals the fragmentation we seem to create.

This is the yearned for in the moments of unsatisfactoriness – yet This-ness is always here.

This is the fusion of observer, observation and observed in a moment of clarity.

This is the agitation in the agitated – and the calm in the peaceful.

This-ness is the essence of happiness, joy without the need for the impression of a past or the projection of a future.

This-ness plays.

This is the eddy currents and whirlpools forming and passing in the stream of wholeness – a timeless journey illuminating its source.

This is the essence of each intimate moment – an endless climax.

This is the arising and passing of TI/ME without separation, effervescently transcendent.

TI/ME lusts to label This, but This cannot be labelled.

There is no way to interpret This, yet This translates itself in all which we are involved.

This nurtures and integrates in a relational moment – interfacing the particular and the whole.

This is intensely calm, like the scintillating midnight forest glow, and the vibrant sound of its trees as they grow.

This is potently dynamic – yet is tranquilly still.

This-ness is shining.

This is the gap between the notes – while the notes amplify the awareness of the gaps.

This is made opaque by the world of things – but in the same instant these things help to illuminate This.

This is the impulse of TI/ME arising – and insight of TI/ME passing.

This gives to all with no need to receive anything in return – empty of TI/ME yet full with the quality of passing.

Whatever manifests, manifests in This, but This never reveals itself in the manifest.

This receives all things without intention – full, yet empty.

This is the knowing in all that is known – nothing yet everything. The experiencing in all that is experienced.

This is the division-less nature of arising and passing – yet when separated by TI/ME is perceived as objects and time.

This-ness is tingling.

This lures the curious to its calm abiding – while offering an intensity of potential.

Concealed in a lonely moment – but is never alone.

Veiled by a lack of conviction – but is itself never in doubt.

This disguises and exposes in the same motion – a paradox of expression.

A dance of dynamic stillness in the midst of stagnation – a transparent secret.

Peaceful yet potent – both calm and intense.

This-ness is joyful.

This illuminates the health beneath the impression of a shadow – the fragments dissolve to reveal they are in essence none other than wholeness itself.

This has no intention other than to reveal itself – the perfection in every imperfection.

This is witnessing and reflecting the dance of the firefly in the forest air and the smell of dung on rotting wood – intimate with all experience.

This is, whether veiled or unveiled – forever scintillating.

This is the gentle whisper of a pregnant universe – coming to be and ceasing to be, vibrating as an expression of wholeness.

This is the touch of the breath,
The experiencing of embodiment,
The potency of presence,
The vitality of vibration,
The free flow of the unhindered felt-sense,
The wholeness of being,
The completeness of now,
This Is.

10.11 Socially reactive versus pro-relational

Currently, there is a promising shift in the way body-based therapists are relating, in an embodied manner, to the conditions presented by various clients. This may be happening, in part, due to understanding the social requirements that a human needs to feel safe. The therapeutic benefits achieved by enhancing social engagement with a client, rather than treating them as a mere bio-mechanical object, are countless. Nevertheless, while this is useful, and indeed commendable, we must be careful not to confuse social engagement with social reactivity.

Social reactivity is where the communication between the therapist and the client remains superficial and follows a theme of socially relevant theatrics to please one another. Such communication avoids the acknowledgement of what is actually being felt by adopting an attitude which avoids external conflict while suppressing internal conflict and following assumed expectations known as the 'fawning response'.[24]

Excessively happy and overly expressive mannerisms are a sure-fire way of bantering a session into superficiality, with limited depth, or even insignificance. If a client is superficially geared up in this way, and we reactively follow suit to fit the skin-deep social appetite, then we are also missing an opportunity to attune with the deeper expressions of health.

However, a therapist who recognizes this social reactivity does not ignore the mirror neurone mimicry, rather they deepen into the subtler felt-sense relationship and help to pave a 'path' for the client to deepen as well.

When a therapist gets wind of a client's subconscious habits they can be aware of their own reactions and empathic responses and can gently taper down any social reactivity while promoting their felt-sense social empathy. This pro-relational social engagement can be achieved by pausing between sentences more and listening to the client with a felt-sense presence of the whole body (calm intensity). Of course, this may not be in line with the subconscious expectations of the client, yet it is, nonetheless, a major ingredient to help open the inherent treatment process at greater depth. The felt-sense of wholeness, still-ness and calm intensity is subtly contagious (in a good way) and the client will invariably settle into a relatively new way of perceiving their body. This is being pro-relational and it comes about by non-doing in an engaged manner.

10.12 Co-regulation versus co-reliance

The human autonomic nervous system receives information from the exteroceptors, interoceptors and the higher tiers of the brain, and responds by telling the body to adopt either one of three survival states, or one of three perceptually safe interaction states. The three survival states comprise of a) mobilisation (fight/flight); b) immobilisation (freeze/flop); or c) pantomime surrender (fawning).[25] The three per-ceived safety states comprise of a) verbal/non-verbal interaction (social engagement); b) play (mental and physical); or c) Intimacy (i.e. sex).

If one of the survival states get stuck in 'on' mode, then the individ-ual's physiology will become more and more dis-regulated. Whereas feeling safe in the presence of another, or others, promotes physiologic co-regulation, which is a wonderful antidote to counter survival states, especially those which have become caught in one or the other (see Appendix 2).

However, depending on a person (or group of people) to establish a balanced physiology will likely reveal an issue at some point. That issue is the one that this book has thus far attempted to explain; if I depend on any 'other' (object, substance, event, etc.) for achieving a felt-sense of safety, then I will concurrently be reliant on the illusion of TI/ME due to it producing the impression of separation.

Yet, perceived safety states which enhance physiologic co-regu-lation, with another or others, are incredible moments for realizing the insight of TI/ME passing and for felt-sense connection to be understood. Therapists who help others achieve this with ease are those who Stephen Porges calls 'super-regulators'. These are individuals who have the capacity to appease another person's unbalanced expressions.

However, it is very common for co-regulatory moments to be missed by the therapist and instead replaced by TI/ME based reactions. Often a therapist who reacts with TI/ME will continue reacting until the chronologic time of the treatment session runs out. It is, therefore, useful for a therapist reacting to TI/ME to start to realize the felt-sense nature of arising and passing in their own body, for example the power of realizing 'This'.[26]

In contemporary psychotherapeutic circles it has become almost vogue for a therapist to talk and move with their client in a safe and fluid manner to help augment the benefits of physiologic co-regulation. This can be very useful to help the client become secure with the idea and initial understanding of feeling safe. However, when co-regulation leads to the client being dependant on the therapist's presence and interaction, rather than accessing their own inherent insight, then after a while such co-regulation techniques will seem artificial, and ultimately dis-satisfying.

Embodied non-doing insight is a great antidote for dissipating co-reliance as the very nature of felt-sense insight simply can't get lost in technique, and projecting to the client the need for perpetual therapeutic support will be seen for what it is. This very insight acts as a boon for all therapists, and their clients, by attaining a felt-sense understanding of TI/ME passing.

A client's perception of being safely engaged in the non-doing presence of a therapist, therefore, helps them to sense co-regulation as an inherently embodied quality rather than forming a projected dependence on the therapist and/or technique to access their health. It is in these moments that a client no longer needs to be identified by their narrative, primed on the premise of trying to survive, and is provided with the quality, safety and freedom of their own inherent embodiment.

10.13 Client resourcing

Now that therapeutic non-doing is acknowledged as both calmly inter-active and intimately alive, we can attend to the relevance of helping to resource the client when and where necessary.

The END therapist is aware that non-doing is *not* a state of being brain dead or just letting things happen in a dissociated manner. To illustrate this metaphorically: without rowing the boat we should just let the wind touch the sails to propel it. Yet, when appropriate, we should also be in a position to steer the boat, fuelled by the insight of also being touched by the wind. In this regard, steering the boat would involve verbally guiding the client towards methods they can use to resource themselves. This may involve reminding the client of their breath and felt-sense perception of their weight, outline, skin sense and internal sense (WOSI[27]), especially if the therapist notices that the client is cycling or drifting in TI/ME. In this way, resourcing may also involve providing the client with ways of de-clutching from agitation or excessive thinking by providing a practice of visualization or imagination.

The calm intensity state of the therapist will help optimize the choosing and relevance of various methods of resourcing. This is be-cause there will be less intention-based distraction coming from the therapist's mind and more guidance from felt-sense insight.

◆ Chapter 11 ◆

The Doing Client

Keep close to nature's heart.

JOHN MUIR

11.1 Falconer and falcon

Until this point we have been exploring intention and non-doing within the therapist and highlighting the prerequisites needed to familiarize, practise and promote the insight of calm intensity and non-doing. Now we shall look at intention and non-doing within the context of a client.

When you contact a client, in the manner we have discussed, then in effect the 'ball is in their court'. They have made the commitment to attend the session and you have made the commitment to invoke calm in-10-city insight. Now they will either let their system display its intelligence or they will resist.

There is an interesting phenomenon which occurs when a falconer trains a falcon. If a falcon falls asleep[1] on the gauntlet[2] of the trainer then when it wakes it will perceive the falconer as an ally and will return after hunting.[3] However, the falcon that remains tense and wary of the trainer during training, even when it knows that there is a source of food, is more likely not to return when it is freed to hunt.

Similarly, a client may use methods to resist the surfacing patterns of experience and opt to remain with the habits that keep experience buried.

Furthermore, a client may exaggerate the overt nature of these habits in order to enhance their sense of identity and distract from any patterns of experience which may be surfacing.

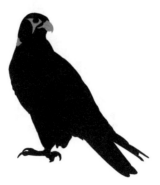

Figure 11.1: Falcon

11.2 Controlling the breath

A client may start to exaggerate their breathing pattern in order to feel the charged arousal of the sympathetic nervous system. Alternatively, a client may start to subconsciously hold their breath to enable dissociation from an environmental stimulus, or experience. Here we are talking about a habit which prevents a pattern of experience from expressing itself.

So, it could be that the result of a pattern expressing itself causes increased ventilation or holding of the breath. In such a case, we are in a position to help if we can discern whether the client's body is expressing itself, or the client is (you guessed it) doing!

When we become aware that it is the client's intention to control the breath then we can attend to this intention by incorporating all the principles outlined in non-doing while touching the client on a relevant region of their body to help increase the awareness of subtle sensations there. For example, non-doing touch at any of the accessory breathing muscles may help balance the subconscious cyclical intention of evoking the sympathetics. Alternatively, non-doing touch at the region of the diaphragm may encourage dissociative breath-holding patterns to dissipate and make way for more functional breathing.

That said, it is better to remain with the contact you have when you notice the client's intentional pattern and wait to find out what non-doing touch can enable from there. If the habit continues, despite this non-doing contact, then utilize the options mentioned.

11.3 Moving the body

It is also common for therapists to encounter a client controlling other areas of their body during a treatment session. For example, a client may intentionally start turning their head or clenching their feet. This can at first be difficult to distinguish between a wilful motor intention and a subconscious pattern of expression. However, a therapist offering embodied non-doing touch will provide the 'insight space' to be able to discern this.

It is better not to talk with clients about their voluntary movements too soon as it may evoke a more covert distraction pattern. Moreover, the client's voluntary body movements might also be a subconscious intention surreptitiously requesting the therapist to do/say something (thus facilitating a distraction in another way).

Engaged non-doing contact, interspersed with an appropriate and timely word or two, encourages the underlying reactive intentions of the client to dissipate and the various physiologic patterns of experience to surface.

If the client's reactive intent does not dissipate, and the body movements continue after a generous period of non-doing contact, then it is generally beneficial to bring in some dialogue to help the client become aware of areas of their body where sensations are not reacted to, and where they can gauge their own interpretation of balance and health.

During such dialogue, it is useful for the therapist to continue with non-doing contact by returning awareness to their own access attention, especially if the sense of calm intensity is lost.

11.4 Subconscious tension

A client firmly holding their body, rather than moving it, may be another manifestation of their intent to feel tension rather than experience unfamiliar patterns, or to prevent them feeling nothing.[4] This kind of tension eases with CITC contact. It doesn't matter whether it eases slowly or quickly, as long as dissociative tendencies are not encouraged. CITC touch encourages integration, so any dissociation tendencies will usually diminish as the treatment continues.

11.5 Asking the therapist to 'focus' on specific areas

A client may present with a directing attitude and try to be in control of where the therapist makes contact. It is of course good to respect this to avoid being perceived as having this very same trait ourselves. Nevertheless, at some point it often proves useful to ask the client to describe the nature of their sensations at an area distant to the locality of contact you have been directed. The client will often mention any number of gross sensations which they perceive (or they may mention the absence of sensations in particular areas). At this point, invite them to persevere by noticing any subtler sensations moving as an under-current to the gross sensations (or seeming absence of sensations). It is interesting how this occupies the client's mind and at the same time causes them to reappraise the perception of their body.[5] In effect, this helps to dissolve the strings of the person pulling the strings.

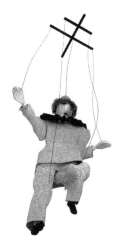

Figure 11.2: Intention of the puppeteer

11.6 Asking the therapist for a wide perceptual field

This is rare in the client setting, but common in undergraduate treatment sessions when students are treating each other. This is because the student being the client can sometimes become informed enough to develop their sensitivity but more often than not lag behind with equanimity and insight.

On occasion, however, a client in the clinic may ask for a wider perceptual field, or use words implying this wish, and when it is provided the client 'goes off with the fairies' (dissociates). This is an important intention to recognize as often the client is in effect asking for permission to fall into a habit of dissociating from the awareness of their body.

When we set up a relational field with a non-doing-based touch (CITC) then we are interacting with the body's intelligence. In this way, we are not denying the tendency for a client's body to dissociate. However, dissociation cannot last for long with such contact. This is because the therapist's calm intensity will be felt by the client, even if their body sensations are not felt. The client will most likely translate the felt-sense the therapist is providing as feeling safe. Gradually this feeling of safety will evolve to feeling sensations, patterns and wholeness in their body and being.

11.7 Talking to distract from deepening

A client can often talk during a session. Sometimes this is to bring the therapist's attention to what they are feeling. However, the client can talk to retain the familiarity of their repetitive thoughts and explicit memories.

If this circumstance is discerned by the therapist then it can prove useful to gently lengthen the period of silence between the time the client stops talking and when you, as the therapist, take over the conversation. The client will generally start to get the gist of silence and stillness in an acceptable way. If questions are posed by the client then try the same approach; increase the length of time you take to answer. In addition to this, it is profoundly useful to stay in contact with the felt-sense of non-doing (CITC). The client will be implicitly learning the language of non-doing in a very palatable way.

11.8 Client transference

The client can potentially react to a therapist, in a manner similar to an early significant figure in their life. This is especially possible when a therapist provides a sense of safety via touch. So an END therapist is wise to be aware of this possibility and notice the cues which suggest a client is reacting in this way. Being aware of this does not require a therapist to then psychologize or change the unfolding transference pattern. A therapist will provide far more benefit for the client by acknowledging the expressions of TI/ME arising in the client's system and provide non-doing felt-sense space for them to unfold.

If the therapist somatically acknowledges the sensations, without countertransference (without reacting to the client's reaction), then insight, of TI/ME passing, will gradually filter into the client's awareness. In other words, when the therapist is aware of felt-sense non-doing in their own body, while acknowledging the client's system, without judgement, labelling, diagnoses and so on, the client gets to experience sensations that would otherwise be inaccessible.

Therapeutic non-doing in this particular instance is very often the missing link required by the client's system to help reintegrate and resource. It is, therefore, useful for the END therapist to be mindful of the huge benefit relational non-doing touch can provide for the well-being of the client. Of course, there will be times when the therapist's awareness is lagging and a level of subconscious somatic countertransference develops. At such times, the therapist may feel sleepy, start yawning, shift their body unexpectedly, develop a headache, cough, get a tense feeling in their muscles or an aching in their joints, feel numb, sexually aroused, nauseous, dizzy and so on. When such unfamiliar session-based feelings arise in the therapist then the felt-sense familiarity of TI/ME passing is the *only* antidote which does not involve suppression or avoidance. In this way, the client does not receive a reaction to their own reactions. It is very likely that they have received reaction to their transference-based reactions on a daily basis, in one way or another, and to be in a relational field which acknowledges without subconscious or conscious countertransference is a game changer for their system to feel more whole.

All that said, it is important to point out that engaged non-doing does not mean that we remain silent and listen to the calm intensity of wholistic passing without ever speaking to the client. It might be relevant, indeed necessary, to ask the client how they are feeling and establish whether they are okay with the feelings that are coming up in them. It can be useful to help them return to the awareness of their body with various simple questions based on the body sensations they are aware of. This can help reorientate the client to the reality of the interaction and serve as a useful reference for the client not to get sucked into a slipstream of reactive tendencies. Still, it is better that the therapist does not get too caught up in their own slipstream of over-guidance, as this prevents the felt-sense insight of TI/ME passing in their own body. When obvious client transference enters the session, the therapist can achieve a tactful dance between relevant doing and non-doing.

11.9 Projecting the therapist as a guru

Transference can also provoke the client to project the therapist as a guru-like figure. The reason for this is when a client's expression of health, balance and sometimes profound systemic shifting occurs, there is an understandable tendency for their mind to want to make sense of it. Sometimes the client won't ask the therapist for an under-standing and instead they deduce the thing that makes most sense. The simplest explanation that a number of clients rest with is that you (the therapist) have the gift of healing and are able to channel energy through your hands.[6]

As complementary as this might at first appear, it is also a potential issue for both the client and the therapist. The more a client projects in this way the more dependent they will become on the therapist to 'heal' them. In essence, this is the same sort of dependence a vehicle owner will have on a mechanic to fix their car. Moreover, as impressions continue to develop in this manner, the more it will divorce the client from potential insight into what is actually occurring. This inevitably impacts on a client's ability to self-regulate and understand the deeper meaning of health.

A further issue, regarding this kind of projection, can occur if a large number of clients are beguiled by the impression of a therapist being a magician. The larger the number of clients who project in this manner, the more likely it is that the therapist will get enticed into believing it themselves. This leads us back to the 'grey zone' issue, and such perspective will be a huge limiting factor for treating with insight.

If anyone reading this is thinking 'Well, a large number of people who want to perceive me as a guru, and follow me like I am the pied piper, will be good for my business', then it may be worthwhile reflecting on the reasons you are inspired by this therapy. END is a deeply genuine therapy which cuts out a lot of the pantomime acts and intentions inherent in many other intention-based therapies. Clients will come to recognize this authenticity, and your reputation as a therapist will attract many people who would otherwise be put off (by inauthenticity).

If the therapist is well versed in their own embodied non-doing felt-sense then the application of techniques is not a problem. Actually, it increases the effectiveness of the technique, regardless of what it is. There are many cases whereby the use of an initial technique is both useful and necessary (as is explained in the next chapter), while it becomes less necessary as non-doing replaces the technique. Techniques can also give the client another focus other than the therapist, which thereby acts as a method preventing the client's deification of the therapist. This subtle dance of technique utilization and cessation is informed by many variables, as will be outlined in Chapter 12.

11.10 Trauma

Having said all this, it must be remembered that it may be relevant to provide a client with appropriate space for their need to 'do', which is different from encouraging the client to avoid arising patterns. This is especially important to acknowledge when a client is presenting with a history of trauma. A client need only be guided to become aware of their distractive tendencies when the therapist has established the client's ability to accommodate the arising of potentially unsettling sensations.

The reason for this is that a traumatized client who halts their reactive tendencies too soon may face arising of memories before they are ready. The following Greek myth may serve as a useful metaphor to help illustrate and understand this better.

Perseus, a demi-god, and son of Zeus and Danae, was set with the seemingly impossible task of slaying the treacherous gorgon Medusa. The problem with this task was that all who had tried to do this previously were turned to stone when they looked into Medusa's eyes (or her sisters, Stheno and Euryale). Fortunately, Perseus was given a heads-up by the goddess Athena and issued with a reflective shield. When confronting Medusa, and her sisters, Perseus tilted the shield so he could see the reflection of the sisters rather than looking directly into their mesmerizing eyes. In this way, he was able to terminate the wicked gorgons and save lots of people from an inevitable fate.

In the same way, if a client is using distraction as a method for not facing intense memories, this should be respected. The client intuitively knows that they will turn to stone (freeze) when they no longer distract from the past experiences, whether explicit or implicit. However, the therapist treating such a client is in a position to apply the appropriate dose and pace needed to craft a process (see following chapter) of not looking directly at the memories, while not avoiding the task required to become embodied.

After this, a client can be appropriately taught how to bring in various felt-sense awareness exercises for themselves, without being overwhelmed. Thus, clients exhibiting patterns of trauma will often benefit remarkably well from this approach, due mostly to the fluid-like safety provided by felt-sense non-doing, and the self-regulatable pacing of any techniques deemed necessary.

◆ EXPERIENTIAL EXERCISE 17

Noticing the client's awareness of passing

- ◆ In pairs, one person is supine on the table (client), one person is at their feet (therapist).

- ◆ Place a simple object (e.g. a ping pong ball) above the client's face, hanging from the ceiling. Or, identify an object such as a lightshade or a mark on the ceiling and position the table in a way that allows the client to be looking directly at it.

- ◆ Go through the SOBA set-up and then touch the client's feet.

- ◆ Be aware of the body expressions, gross and subtle.

- ◆ After a couple of minutes, ask the client to look at the object above them and 'visually absorb' the image, without analysing or evaluating it, for one minute.

- ◆ Tell them to close their eyes and ask them if they are aware of the impression of the object in their mind's eye. If they are not aware of it, ask them to open their eyes and look at the image for a further 30 seconds.

- ◆ Keep repeating this until there is an impression of the object in the client's mind.

- ◆ Ask the client to notice the process of the mind-object dissolving at the same time as noticing sensations in the body dissolving.

- ◆ How is the felt-sense different (for you as the therapist) when the client is noticing the dissipation of mind-object and sensation?

CLINICAL NOTE

This can be a useful dialogue and process to help a client sense the impermanent characteristic of TI/ME and sensation.

It is especially useful when a client is presenting with habits, tendencies and intentions that are preventing subtler patterns of experience from expressing fully.

It is like offering the essence of the focusing technique without the trappings of getting caught in a method.

Chapter 12

Cranioga

Yoga is the progressive settling of the mind into silence. When the mind has settled, we are established in our essential nature, which is unbounded consciousness. Our essential nature is usually overshadowed by the activity of the mind.

PATANJALI

12.1 Cranioga: process of intentional attention leading to non-doing

'Client-based biodynamic craniosacral and yoga therapy emphasizing therapeutically engaged non-doing (TEND)' is a long-winded name, so the term cranioga was coined to make it easier for the tongue. Cranioga is not just another hybrid distortion of yoga attempting to appeal to the contemporary memes of modern minds. Nor is it intended to be a didactic process blinkered by the confines of 'orthodox' yoga. It is, however, a genuine inquiry of relevant resources which serve to catalyse body awareness and insight in the client. The mind often requires excuses to keep it occupied (focused) while being able to appreciate the passing nature of TI/ME.[1] When the mind is tamed and sharpened, in this manner, it will start to illuminate the existence of subtle intentions residing in the body-mind, which unnoticed cause tension but when realized provide release and vitality.

A great ocean of health is waiting to express itself and all it requires is the presence of engaged non-doing.

Prior to helping a client, it is vital to help oneself. This is why the majority of the book has been on the need for a therapist to access the interfacing quality of calm intensity and be affected by the insight it provides.

Accessing calm intensity, by realizing the components of calm in-10-city, or the four chambers of non-doing, or the five factors of insight, helps to reference where one is at during personal END practice and while treating a client. This is not theoretical, it is real-time felt-sense referencing. However, the mind can yearn for a simple theoretical breakdown of what will help optimize the client's expression of health. So here it is.

The therapist learns to access and embody seven fundamental 'therapist-specific' qualities to help the client. These are:

1. Learning to touch into the earth to help ground oneself and help to ground another.

2. Learning to establish a felt-sense of the body fluids in one's self and another.

3. Noticing the subtle transmutation which occurs when tendencies, identification, memories and expectations (TI/ME) are surrendered to their nature of 'passing' rather than the mind's repetition of them. The felt-sense of passing, in biodynamic craniosacral therapy, is called 'potency'.

4. Developing an ability to be aware of the inherent inclination the body has to return to balance when given the right touch and space.

5. Realizing that felt-sense space is energy and potential, rather than conceptual emptiness – it is indeed empty of TI/ME but it is full of vibrant vitality and potential.

6. Realizing that when there is a felt-sense of TI/ME passing there is also a relational field of understanding which is no longer limited by the confines of separation-based thinking. This is here called 'insight'.

7. Letting the permeation of insight develop a felt-sense of wholeness while acknowledging the practical necessity of being able to isolate and identify where necessary.

The resourced and insightfully inspired END therapist will be able to approach the client, with the awareness of these seven TEND qualities checked, so that cranioga treatment can begin with optimal effect.

So, having said that, we will now delve into the treatment process overview. Cranioga is a form of restorative yoga helping to reaccess the awareness of subtle sensations of the body. It potentially consists of 12 integrative and progressive phases, including: assessment, postural balancing, breath-work and self-regulation. These are key aspects of the process which promote and encourage a sense of embodiment in the client, rather than dissociation.

Having said that, it is non-doing (in the context outlined in this book) which is the major 'ingredient' that is embodied by the therapist throughout the treatment.

Other phases include the instruction of gentle stimulation aware-ness, which can vary from an initial visualization, to tapping relevant areas of the body, to becoming aware of the stimulation caused by air touching the skin when breathing without effort. Other forms of gentle stimulation awareness involve the expression of various emotional gestures, for example those mimicking openness, friendship and ease.

Specific postures are taught to help address asymmetries caused by autonomic nervous system imbalance and are incorporated with physiologic reasoning, rather than asking a client to mimic a pose from a textbook or to try and look cool.

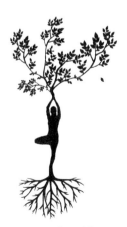

Figure 12.1: Postures to connect earth and heaven and optimize the midline

Breath-work helps a client to increase their embodiment, sensitivity and the willingness to let go, if practised appropriately. The therapist can then facilitate postures and breathing patterns which help to evoke a neurogenic release (which often gets primed following applicable breath-work). The body releases tension in this manner when it is no longer being directed by subconscious reactivity, such as defensive muscular contractions or repetitive nerve impulses.

Preparing the body-mind with breath-work and encouraging spontaneous neurogenic release are the ultimate prerequisites for the access attention often known as *pran-ayama*.[2] *Pran-ayama* is awareness of the natural breath (i.e. without control), which, when observed without intention, but with attention, unveils the subtler body sensations (*pratyahara*). Once a client has become familiar with *pran-ayama*, or any other relevant attention which provides a sense of the body's subtle expressions, then their system usually feels safe like a potent flowing river, and is ready for 'relational touch', the same way an embryo feels resourced with potency and ready to receive the world.

The embryonic intelligence of the body is a dance of the internal fluid expressions free from restrictive patterns of experience. Being aware of this is in itself insight, and is a realization that the embryologic body intelligence is accessible, albeit as a very subtle expression. Actually, the only reason it does not appear to be accessible is due to it being overshadowed by tendencies, impressions, memories and expectations. When insight unfolds, a tangible understanding of what relationship and nature really are becomes clear. This is a flow of connection beyond the constraints of fear and fragmentation. In other words, it is an antidote to the limitations we have been coerced into believing, both consciously and subconsciously.

No lasting antidote will be found by incorporating the opposite to something, for instance gravitating to something we like in favour of something we do not like. It may be practically useful in many cases, but the deep yearning for a sense of stillness, vitality and balance will continue. Suppressing a negative thought, emotion or sensation, and directing preference to what is perceived as positive, merely forms a subconscious shadow of further dissatisfactoriness, which will need to be dealt with at some point if the yearning for stillness, vitality and balance is to be acknowledged. However, insight, which is not born from the duality of thought, shines a light which has no opposite, and therefore no subconscious duality-based reaction is formed.

So, the cranioga process provides a client with a sense of agency and begins with intention (desire to change something); it then transitions to attention, and develops to intention-free awareness (insight), which is being present with change itself. This last phase is embodied non-doing – the 'END'.[3]

12.2 Cranioga treatment

Assessment

Every nanometre of the body is affected by the autonomic nervous system (ANS). When an individual's breathing rhythm is controlled by an activated sympathetic nervous system (SNS), the diaphragm, intercostal and accessory breathing muscles will contract and relax to induce and sustain the amplified ventilation of the lungs. When increased breathing rhythms like this continue over a long period of time the muscles controlling the lungs will eventually become overwhelmed, and the connective tissue supporting the muscles will tighten. This occurs to reduce energy expenditure by mimicking and thus supporting the contraction phase of the muscles.

Other than the diaphragm, the majority of isotonically activated respiratory muscles primed by the SNS are the intercostal muscles, which elevate, expand and retract the ribs and accessory breathing muscles, which act as rib elevators and depressors. In addition to this, spinal extensors resist thoracic flexion to enhance inhalation and thus increase oxygen intake.

CLINICAL NOTE

It is useful for the therapist to note the specific anatomic location of these muscles, especially the spinal extensor muscles, as this helps to ascertain what position will be most beneficial to help release tightness. The spinal extensor muscles are posterior to the mid-coronal plane of the body and are the muscles/connective tissue which we stretch while performing flexion postures. When a client gently stretches these muscles, while lengthening their exhalatory breath followed by a brief pause at the end of the out-breath (*bahir-kumbhaka*), then a release of any stored tension can often be observed or felt as a slight twitch or even a tremor. When the therapist does not react with worry or evasively ignore these physiologic expressions, as has been explained, then the client is implicitly getting the thumbs up that this is a natural and useful somatic release. Non-reactive touch or presence is often all that is needed. It may also be that the expressions are much more subtle, yet still felt by the therapist, perhaps as a fluid flow or maybe the tingling sense of arising and passing, in which case the same applies.

The 'apprehension reflex'[4] is an SNS primed reaction causing an alert recoil and temporary immobilization. This is similar to the sudden cessation of motion which occurs when the music stops in a game of musical chairs, which at the same time results in either a gasp and re-tention of inhaled air, or a sudden exhalation with concurrent restraint from inhaling. In other words, this reaction causes a momentary accentuation of filling or emptying the lungs. This type of breath re-tention will activate isometric contraction of either the thoracic spine extensors or flexors, and, if sustained or repeatedly activated, will result in the formation of tension and tightness in related myofascia. As a consequence, the SNS will be prompted into 'on mode', causing an amplified breathing pattern, which is one of the most obvious signs a therapist can observe. When there is a reactive cycle of TI/ME feeding the ANS, the SNS 'on mode' will likely become chronic. As mentioned, a client's activated breathing pattern is generally quite apparent while they are being assessed, but do remain aware of the habit a client has of holding their breath; this is harder to notice than the panting nature of hard breathing.

CLINICAL NOTE

If the therapist has the right devices and/or skills in the clinic then the client's heart rate variability can be assessed. The effect of the client's breath on their heart rate will generally be less coherent with chronic on-mode SNS activation. Still, if such devices and skills are not present, then assessing the tempo and retention of the client's breath is a straightforward and demonstrable sign of chronic SNS activation.

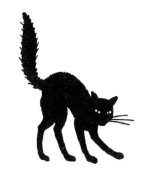

Figure 12.2: Apprehension reflex

The parasympathetic nervous system (PNS) affects the respiratory muscles in a very different way to the SNS. In a socially engaged and/ or perceptibly safe environment, the activation of the PNS will inhibit the autonomic contraction of the accessory breathing muscles and regulate the breathing rhythm in a calm and sustainable manner. The PNS will continue by promoting relaxed diaphragm activity, with moderate intercostal work, and will relinquish the need for any other accessory breathing muscular activity. The PNS-regulated breathing rhythm will automatically slow and lengthen exhalation, which, over time, increases the carbon dioxide in the body tissues ready for an effective exchange with oxygen from the blood when inhalation increases again. This helps an individual feel sufficiently resourced to engage at a social level and to become more aware of TI/ME passing when the environment is appropriate (see Appendix 2).

However, a contrasting physiologic presentation unfolds when the perceived environment poses a significant life-threatening situation. This results in the ANS overriding a coherently balanced heart beat in addition to overriding the SNS and its effect on mobilizing the body. This is a physiologic state called 'hypertonic immobility', which isometrically contract the major trunk and abdomen flexor muscles helping to protect many of the vital organs.

CLINICAL NOTE

These are the same muscles which we primarily stretch while performing extension and twisting postures of the trunk, and to good effect when the environment feels safe enough to remind the body to release these muscles.

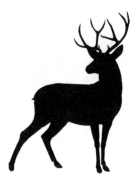

Figure 12.3: Hypertonic immobility response

If the hypertonic immobility state is sustained over long periods of time, and/or there is additional stress or trauma imposed on the system, or the unfolding situation seems hopeless from a survival perspective, then there is a possibility that the body will become limp and exhausted. This is the body adopting a physiologic state called *hypotonic* immobility (inhibited muscle activation due to increased dorsal-vagal input). When this survival response is adopted much of the sub-diaphragmatic smooth muscle function shuts down and the organs become torpid. Also, any air breathed during this exhausted, and likely dissociated, state will mostly fill and empty very shallowly, and occasionally not at all. Often humans are able to just about function while being chronically caught in such survival states, but this comes at a physiologic cost, causing organs and the nervous system to operate suboptimally.

Considering all this, it is important not to forget that the most valuable aspect of the assessment is the non-doing acknowledgement you, the END therapist, are providing while assessing. A client's system, acknowledged in this way, is given the 'energy' and confidence to seek balance. It is good to keep remembering this, because helping a client's body to find balance and re-associate is not in essence a technique. Any techniques used are mostly to placate a client's mind enough for the client to feel heard and met, in a relevant way, at least enough initially for him or her to access their felt-sense via the prism of a logical rationale.

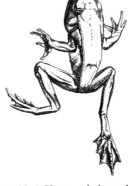

Figure 12.4: Hypotonic immobility

Disordered breathing patterns subconsciously substantiate the existence of TI/ME. In other words, a disordered breathing pattern supports the impression of a permanent separate self and the fragmented perspective that goes with it. This perspective also correlates with physiologic burden, at least as far as energy expenditure goes. Inversely, a balanced calm breathing pattern exposes the reality of TI/ME passing and reveals this as a potent quality with no permanent content. This provides an entirely different perspective of self, one which dissolves the physiologic burden of TI/ME. Awareness of this is awareness of awareness being aware. In other words, it is presence itself shimmering in its reflection. There is no narcissism with such awareness, as it is realized that there is no individual, permanent mirror, and therefore no 'I'. This is entirely different from being in a state of dissociation.

When there is a feeling of safety during the practice of being still and alert[5] then the unique hybrid combined activation of both dorsal and ventral aspects of the vagus nerve provide a 'state' of immobilization without fear.[6] Familiarization of the ventral vagal activation in this way can then permeate into social engagement and activities which involve mobilization with a sense of safety, such as sport. An individual who has become familiar with enhancing ventral vagal activity mostly demonstrates a pliant breathing pattern.

CLINICAL NOTE

So, observing the rhythm and habits of a client's breathing at the start of a session helps us to establish what setting the ANS is tuned to, and from there we can apply a relevant intention/ attention/non-doing approach. A client's posture, gesticulations, eye contact, fidgeting, concentration and so on can also provide further clues as to how much intention, attention or non-doing is appropriate.

Evaluation of 'dosage' and pacing

After the assessment has helped the therapist evaluate and sense the client's autonomic nervous system, the application of treatment can be tailored to suit the needs of the client's body. For example, for a client with an agitated nervous system, the postures recommended by the therapist will involve a greater degree of calming flexion postures to begin with. For those who are exhibiting an excessive fawning[7] response, the prescription of gentle yet attentive breaths and/or sensory awareness techniques can be useful to begin with, to save the client from building up too much ANS duress.

Gentle stimulation awareness (including *mudras*)

Gentle invigoration techniques applied to various areas of the client's body helps to wake their system up to the environment and become more aware of sensations expressing themselves in the body. The stimulation needs to be gentle and simple – so gentle in some cases that visualization is all that is needed. This can be the image of the client being in a calm location such as a field with a gently flowing stream. Gradually guide the client by adding more colour or objects to the imagined picture. It is better, in the long run, to keep visualizations brief. This is to save the tendencies of the mind over-indulging in this aspect of the process. Nevertheless, when significant trauma is part of the client's history, then more time might be required for this aspect. Progression from visualization might include gestures (*mudras*) using a part of the body such as the face or hands, or perhaps the whole body. In this instance, it is best to ask the client to become aware of an emotion and express it with any gesture which feels most relevant. This activates the connection between the emotions and the body. Certain gestures can also calm or energize the body.[8]

An additional way of bringing in gentle stimulation is to ask the client to blow through relaxed closed lips three or four times. Such blowing makes a fluttering sound as the air flaps the lips up and down. After the stimulation, ask the client to relax and become aware of the subtle sensations expressing themselves at the lips. Then invite the client to notice if the sensations spread to the cheeks, the face, the head and perhaps the whole body.

Another useful region to stimulate is the nails of the fingers of both hands.[9] This can be done by touching the nails of opposite hands together and rubbing them for a minute at the level of the heart. After the client has finished rubbing the nails, ask them to become aware of the tingling sensations presenting in the fingers, hands, arms and whole body.

Figure 12.5: Fingernail rubbing

To gently stimulate the lower aspect of the body you can suggest the client walks barefoot on various, palatable, surfaces and again bring attention to the subtle nature of the sensations that show themselves when the client stands still.

In addition to this, if the therapist needs to become more embodied during a treatment session, it is best not to adopt the examples outlined above. Actually, END therapists do not need to, especially as we get more and more versed with the subtle stimulus which is happening all of the time; for example, the stimulus of the breath touching the inner nostrils and skin of the upper lip. The more sensitivity a therapist develops, the more the subtle stimulation of sound or light vibration will be enough to help embodiment happen automatically. The only issue in this case will be to remember to bring awareness to these areas when it is needed.

Relevant postures (*asana*)

Specific postures, based on the client's presenting ANS expression, are extremely helpful for encouraging suitable ANS tone and balance. It is not the mechanical stretch component of an *asana* that helps release overly tense or tight tissue, it is the awareness of TI/ME passing, and a sense of space, which resets the ANS. The awareness of space and insight of TI/ME passing can be increased by teaching the client how to breathe relevantly in the specific postures. Refer back to access attention for the various postures and breathing patterns which help balance the mind and increase the awareness of the body.

The incorporation of challenge, by guiding the client into various challenging but not forceful body postures, helps a client's impression of certain structural limits dissolve into the expression of 'potency' (the perception of TI/ME passing). This helps to open new somatic possibilities regarding function and capacity. It is common, however, at least in contemporary *asana* practice, for people to force their body into positions they are not ready for. This causes unnecessary strain and prevents the relaxed awareness required to perceive the subtler sensations. For example, in extension postures there should be a subtle but distinct sense of energizing; in flexion a sense of calming; in rotation a sense of expansion and a sense of fluidity, and so on. Therefore, if an individual is not calmly aware of these subtle sensations, the *asana* practice is merely a mechanical endeavour, which is not what many original yogis, such as Patanjali,[10] wished to convey.

Another very simple and yet extremely effective method of posture adoption are the salamander postures presented by Stanley Rosenberg. Easily adopted head, neck and trunk postures combined with various lateral eye movements can 'reveal' hidden hypertonic immobility patterns in the body. When these postures are sustained and relaxed into for a certain duration, the dorsal vagus circuit switches to a ventral vagus circuit and the individual will often let out a sigh/deep breath, yawn or swallowing action.

A therapist can subtly adopt micro-postures during a treatment session to help balance a conflicting disposition. When a therapist is well versed in the physiologic effects of various postures then a very tiny shift in position is often all that is needed to titrate into a balanced state of physiologic presence. However, a therapist who changes their posture in this manner is not adopting it to avoid what is being expressed in their body; rather it is to help settle/balance their system enough to utilize access attention (see Chapter 7).

The infinitesimally small shift adopted by the therapist should not be enough to be noticed by the client. In this way, it will often be enough to remind both the therapist and the client's body of balance. Incidentally, barely one or two of these shifts are needed during a treatment session as one deepens with this practice.

Stretch/engage/release

This is a principal inclusion which can bring about a significant transformation in body awareness and relaxation.[11] To apply this most effectively, ask the client to relax halfway through a specific posture, then instruct them to contract the same muscle they were previously stretching (they will likely need your anatomical guidance for this). The contraction should be sustained for ten to fifteen seconds, at 50 per cent of their maximal effort. After releasing the contraction, ask the client to take a deep breath in and out, then continue by adopting the original posture, which will probably be deeper than it was before the contraction. More importantly, it will likely increase the client's felt-sense engagement of at least one area of their body.

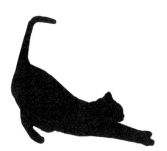

Figure 12.6: Stretching cat

Breath-work

Breath-work builds on the specific postures which have been practised for the relevant duration and tailored for their individual benefits. Breath-work is not *pran-ayama* – which is non-control of the natural breath while observing it. Instead, breath-work is where there is intentional control of the breath in a manner which evokes either the sympathetic or parasympathetic aspects of the autonomic nervous system. The specific technique is taught to help further balance the client's system and act as a 'primer' to enter *pran-ayama* (non-doing breath). All the while, the END therapist remains as aware as possible of their own natural breath, be it fast, moderate or slow.

The really simple yet useful regulation of breath is gradually extending the out-breath compared to the in-breath. This helps to increase vagal tone, which will be of benefit for a vast majority of the human population.

Pandiculation (helping to establish *pratyahara*)

Pandiculation is the word used to describe the autonomic nervous system's way of waking the sensorimotor nerves, and their surrounding tissues, to either prepare us for movement or to enable the release of stored tension.

We all know how it feels as it is the unchoreographed stretch we often do first thing in the morning, yawning with an outstretched limb or two. Pandiculation sends informative biofeedback to our somatic nervous system, letting it know the area and level of subconscious tightness and contraction held in our connective and contractile tissue. It especially helps to regulate the gamma neurone feedback loop connecting the nervous system to the muscles. Foetuses regularly pandiculate in the womb, which can be visibly observed, demonstrating how deeply ingrained and primal this response is.

During treatment sessions, a client may present with involuntary movements, twitches, flickers, stretches which come out of the blue, yawns and so on. These are visible movements of the body and are generally not brought about by intention. Actually, these overt expressions are visible releases of TI/ME and are, therefore, a somatic expression of subconscious intent dissipating.

A therapist who provides non-doing touch doesn't react to these pandiculatory movements. This results in the client feeling safe for them to continue. Their system is getting the 'it's okay to express this' thumbs up. If a client needs to have some verbal confirmation that it is normal for the body to express in this way then keep dialogue brief, as less talk will help their system to unfold further.

Non-doing releases tremors and flow (helping to establish *pratyahara*)

This describes the spontaneous neurogenic tremors and flow states[12] produced by the body when it is given the right cues. It is different from pandiculatory release movements, although, like pandiculatory movements, it also helps the client to become more balanced and internally aware (*pratyahara*). This is because central pattern generators (CPGs) in the central nervous system (CNS) are activated causing an overt rhythmic tremor motion which is not retrained by the motor cortex of the brain. This means that there is an autonomic rhythmic output (release) with an absence of voluntary somatic output (control).

The therapist can encourage these movements by asking the client to adopt certain jaw, neck, arm, lower back and hip positions with the inclusion of certain methods of breath regulation. As mentioned, such therapist-guided facilitation is only necessary in specific circumstances.

Incidentally, the language the therapist uses to help the client understand varying aspects of this process is a skill which can be tuned via supervision, relevant courses and...experience.

Access attention (*pran-ayama* and *dharana*)

Access attention for the therapist has been described in detail throughout this book. In order to guide a client, the therapist should ascertain the client's propensities and decide on the most useful access attention method for them. This may be asking the client to visually focus on an object and notice the image dissipate with closed eyes, or striking a small gong and asking the client to listen to the 'sound of passing', and so on. The most universal propensity for clients to access insight is the touch of the natural breath (*pran-ayama*). It is also great for preventing a client who is starting to dissociate from their body.

Pran-ayama develops naturally following on from the previous inclusions. The client's awareness of their own natural breathing joins the therapist's awareness of the natural breath. At this point, harmony has begun and the expression of the client's subtler sensations will undoubtedly start to be illuminated by their awareness. It is useful to draw the client's attention to the touch of their breath in or below their nostrils. They will then be able to add an element of progression by lengthening the duration they are able to remain aware of the natural breath without being distracted. However, measuring duration is not as important as the client adopting a regular practice in this regard.

During *pran-ayama*, a number of somatic releases might unfold and, as long as they are not intentional, the client's awareness will deepen with the insight of TI/ME passing. Having said that, if a client is periodically controlling their body out of habit, after the *pran-ayama* has begun, then it can be useful to orchestrate a neurogenic tremor in the client by asking the client to adopt specific postures and breathe in a particular way. It is beyond the scope of this book to elaborate on this further due to the specificity of such inclusion. Please visit www.cranioga.com for courses that provide guidance and more information regarding this.

Pran-ayama, therefore, helps the client to get a feel for the access attention anchor. However, it might be more relevant for the client to be guided to other specific areas such as the manubrium or below the navel (lower *tan tien*). Once a client has reached this level of awareness the therapist might notice that one of the senses is more sensitive and non-reactive, for example the hearing sense, whereby subtle sound can act as the anchor for access attention.

Client receiving END touch (relational touch – biodynamic craniosacral therapy)

After establishing access attention and embodying the insight of TI/ME passing there is often no more habitual doing that the client needs or wishes to partake in. At this point, the therapist can make contact at relevant areas of the body while treating with embodied non-doing touch, in the manner which has been explained throughout this book.

The client most often lies in the supine position (*shavasana*) and the therapist will be guided by the client's body, while acting as an END reference for the client's body to feel confident enough to reveal itself. By this point, the supine position is often ideal as it no longer mimics the positions feeding back the need for protection, such as the side-lying foetal position, or dissociation, such as the lying prone position.

The natural 'progression' from the start of the cranioga process to *pran-ayama* includes the development of insight. Pandiculation and neurogenic release can occur at any point during the process, but usually when *pran-ayama* begins. The patterns of experience, which release at these points of the process, provide the client with deeper insight into the passing of TI/ME. It is useful here for the therapist to explain what is happening or has happened. However, this is not a necessity in order for insight to deepen. Actually, the insight will deepen as *pran-ayama* continues and the felt-sense awareness of sensations arising and passing occurs in a sustained manner without distraction (*dharana*). Meditation, in the true sense of that word, follows this insight – this is *dhyana*.

At some point the client's body will seem fluidly amorphous and much more connected to the environment and nature in general. This is not a state of dissociation from the body,[13] it is actually the client's body becoming more present as their insight deepens. So, the fluid feel is an expression of the client's presence as well as their insight of TI/ME passing becoming more established. This insight is not another impression or perspective based on duality. Rather, it is a realization which is both conscious of the relative world (duality) and its relevance, while being conscious of the absolute wholeness of non-duality.

Self-regulation (*dhyana* with insight) (calm in-10-city)

These final two stages are for the client who has established access attention and has a desire to help others benefit from what they have benefited from. In effect, they are transitioning the emphasis of being a client/student to primarily being an END therapy student. So, the last two stages are only for clients who have the genuine motivation to help others and are balanced enough to do so.

Calm in-10-city, as discussed earlier in the book, is the term describing the break down of ten qualities ('ingredients') which provide a felt-sense interface between duality and non-duality. This interface opens to the insight of TI/ME passing and is the 'bedrock' of engaged non-doing. A client/student who is able to access and understand this interface is now a person able to fully resource/regulate themselves and, potentially, help transmute the effects of TI/ME in another. In other words, they are ready to learn to become a therapist themselves – if this is their inclination.

Client/student offering END touch

The ability to provide relational touch could be regarded as the crescendo of the process, as the client has embodied the insight sufficiently to be a student wishing to learn to help others. If their desire is to authentically offer the insight they have embodied, then the therapist should evaluate whether the client is truly in a position which others will benefit from. Otherwise it is more appropriate to finish the process with a client receiving END touch. Therefore, the END therapist will only mention the last two stages to the client if it seems relevant. Even then it will be recommended that the client only treats members of their family or close friends. After some time, the client may feel drawn to join a cranioga or biodynamic craniosacral therapist training (www.cranioga.com or www.bodyintelligence.com) where they can learn the skills necessary to treat people other than their family and friends.

12.3 Cranioga process in a nutshell

- Above all else, the therapist is in touch with their own calm intensity. The therapist treats and assesses the client while in touch with their own 'calm in-10-city', or five insight characteristics, or four chambers of non-doing (whichever works best).

- Assessment of the client's breath, posture and overall ANS expression.

- Dosage and pacing evaluation and implementation based on the finding from the assessment.

- Gentle stimulation guidance to help the client wake awareness of their subtle body sensations.

- Stretch/engage/release education introduced where relevant to help unearth the sensitivity of various areas of the body, especially those areas suspected to be in a state of fragmented dissociation.

- Relevant postures relating to the client's presentation. This is the part of the process which helps to first balance the client's ANS.

- Breath-work to establish a deeper and longer-lasting balance of the client's ANS.

- The education of *pran-ayama* is incorporated so the client can witness the inherent intelligence of the body and understand how important it is to periodically let go of habitual intention and be in awe of the body's ability to realign and refresh itself – to be aware and non-reactive during the moments of rebalancing.

- It is at this point that the therapist can establish whether a specific area of sensation awareness is better sensed elsewhere or whether the access attention needs more subtle appreciation, such as acknowledging light, sound and so on.

- The therapist notices the pandiculation-based expressions of the client's body and reassures the client that these are normal and useful to help the body re-establish its wholistic felt-sense nature and fluid/potency flow. A therapist sensing their own flow at this point can help the client to overcome any intransigent resistance preventing the flow expression.

- The therapist notices the neurogenic tremors which sometimes present during a session and reassures the client that these are natural expressions of the body which help restore and integrate the physiology. If the client is caught in a control or freeze cycle then it can be useful to guide the client through specific postures and breathing methods to help encourage a neurogenic release.

- Relational touch is best applied from the stage of *pranayama*. It generally unearths deeper patterns of experience. Relational touch reveals the deep patterns of experience held in their body, which are often the reason for a client's unbalanced system. It is good to reassure the client that letting these patterns arise and noticing them pass can engender a new lease of life and vitality. This reassurance will mostly be achieved through engaged non-doing contact (END touch), that is, the therapist being aware of TI/ME passing and not needing to say anything. This is the most effective aspect of an END therapist's treatment, as the client themselves will also start to become aware of what it feels like to be in a 'state' of engaged non-doing and become more and more familiar with the potency and sense of wholeness it provides.

NB: Despite the outlined cranioga process being a concise and slip-streamed option to help optimize and balance a client's autonomic nervous system, please note that any bodywork therapy can be applied alongside the END therapy principles. It is the engaged non-doing (relational) touch which is the game changer, and principles are for the *therapist* to embody. Thereby the process of therapeutic intervention can be applied (if appropriate), and eventually relinquished (when appropriate). The major difference from conventional intention-based therapy is that when an intervention is applied it will now be fuelled by 'insightful doing' rather than 'TI/ME fuelled doing'.

As such, the interventions used are both an excuse for the client to feel met,[14] and a way of helping to balance their autonomic nervous system. This helps the client to appreciate and correlate their perspective of what is 'wrong' with them, with what the therapist is offering.

So, it is important to progress this process in a reasoned fashion and with appropriate intentional intervention at the right time. But it is equally, if not more, important for the therapist to establish calm intensity in themselves, so that intention manifests and dissolves when and where relevant.

◆ Chapter 13 ◆

Loving Presence

Love is the whole thing.

We are only the pieces.

RUMI

13.1 Insightful love versus conjured love

Once calm intensity has opened the insight of non-duality, intent comes from a source free from conditioning. Such intent is 'ground intention'. It is from this source that vibrant thought manifests from insight. Thoughts of this nature are infused with kindness, love and altruism, naturally emitting joy like perfume is emitted from a flower. Thought, in this instance, is a potency expression, rather than an echo of habit, which is free from the content of TI/ME. Thoughts, which are free from being conditioned by TI/ME, are known in the Pali language as the *brahmaviharas*, a series of four foundational Buddhist virtues and meditation practices designed to cultivate them. In English, *brahmavihara* translates to 'divine abode'.

An END practitioner may find it useful to acknowledge the 'scent' of potency within the treatment room, by noticing the vibration which occurs during insight-derived transmutation. This vibration is in the air and walls of the room and permeates everything with a perfume of sorts. Awareness of this 'perfume' enables the therapist to be deeply connected to a form of *brahmavihara* meditation, without even trying. This meditation has been talked about and formulated into a variety of differing techniques for centuries, especially in certain Buddhist traditions. The method of these meditations is outlined below. However, it is good to appreciate that if the insight of non-duality is not present, then such meditations are mere rituals. In which case, such ritual will do little more than calm the mind into a pattern of joy (Pli: *piti*; Skt: *priti*), which is of course wonderful to promote, but will still be under the dominant influence of TI/ME.

Lao-tzu alludes to this in Chapter 18 of the *Tao Te Ching*:

> When the great Tao is forgotten, 'goodness' and 'piety' appear.
>
> When the body's intelligence declines, 'cleverness' and 'knowledge' step forth.
>
> When there is no peace in the family, 'filial piety' begins.
>
> When the country falls into chaos, 'patriotism' is born.

In other words, by forgetting our original nature, intention to change the presenting situation takes over. By replacing our original nature with the idea of change, rather than feeling it, we rely more and more on intention, which will conjure 'love', 'compassion', 'goodness' and so on devoid of insight. As a result, there is potential for this to further exacerbate the forgetting of our original nature. This does not mean we need to vanquish joy, as when it is not dependent on TI/ME it is the essence of our original nature – awareness, equanimity, love and joy are not different here.

When intention to invoke the *brahmaviharas* is 'touched' by non-doing then intention passes and, as a result, thought is now fuelled by insight.

The four sections that follow are the traditionally applied intentional approaches of loving appreciation, compassion, empathetic joy and equanimity.

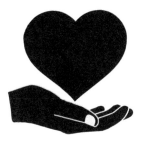

Figure 13.1: Heartful hand

13.2 *Mettā* (loving appreciation)[1]

Mettā meditation, often called loving kindness meditation, is the practice concerned with the cultivation of *mettā*, also known as benevolence, kindness and amity. Here it will be referred to as loving appreciation. The practice generally consists of silent repetitions of phrases such as 'may you be happy' or 'may you be free from suffering', for example directed at a person who, depending on tradition, may or may not be internally visualized. This is obviously a form of directed intention. An important prerequisite, therefore, is to have the intention come from thought fuelled by insight rather than TI/ME.

◆ EXPERIENTIAL EXERCISE 18

Loving appreciation
Mettā

People often find it challenging to direct loving appreciation to themselves. We may feel that we are unworthy, or that it's egotistical, or that we shouldn't be happy when other people are suffering. So rather than start loving appreciation practice with ourselves, which is traditional, it may be more useful to start with those we most naturally love and care about. One of the beautiful principles of compassion and loving appreciation practice is that we start where it is most palatable, where it's easiest – where it works. We open our heart, in a natural unforced way, then direct our loving appreciation to the areas in our own being where it is easy to be appreciated and then gently to areas where it's more difficult.

◆ First, sit comfortably and at ease, with your eyes closed. Sense yourself seated here in this incredible mystery of human life. Take your seat in the paradox of calm intensity, a place halfway between heaven and earth. Then bring a kind attention to yourself, including your tendencies, impressions, sensations, feelings, emotions and ideations. Feel your body grounded and your breath breathing naturally.

◆ Think of someone you care about and perhaps love deeply. Then let natural phrases of good wishes for them come into your mind, heart and being. Phrases can vary, but can include: 'May you be safe and protected', 'May you be healthy, whole and strong', and 'May you be truly happy and peaceful.' These are the traditional ones, but any heartfelt words can replace these.

◆ Then let your mind source the image of a second person you care about and express the same good wishes and intentions towards them.

◆ Next, imagine that these two people, whom you care for and love, are reciprocally offering you their loving appreciation. Picture how they look at you with authentic caring and love as they say: 'May you too be safe and protected. May you be healthy and strong. May you be truly happy.'

◆ With an open heart, accept the good wishes they are offering and receive the vibrations of their loving kindness. Sometimes people place their hand on their heart or a relevant place on their body as they repeat the phrases: 'May I be safe and protected. May I be healthy and strong. May I be truly happy.'

◆ With the same heartfulness, let your eyes open, look around the room, and offer your loving appreciation to everyone around you. Feel how connecting it is to spread the field of loving appreciation. It can be felt, even though many may not be aware of it.

◆ Now think of yourself as a rotating light, spreading the light of loving appreciation around your city, around the country, around the world, even to faraway stars. Think, 'May all beings far and near, all beings young and old, beings in every direction, be held in great loving appreciation. May they be safe and protected, may they express health and be strong, may they be truly happy.'

13.3 *Karuṇā* (compassion)

Karuṇā is the second foundational pillar of the *brahmaviharas*. The Pali commentaries distinguish between *karuṇā* and *mettā* in the following complementary manner: *karuṇā* is the desire to remove harm and suffering from others, while *mettā* is the desire to enhance the well-being and happiness of others. The 'gross hindrance' of *karuṇā* is cruelty, a mind state which is in opposition to compassion, and one which is formulated by TI/ME. The 'subtle hindrance' quality, which superficially resembles *karuṇā* but is in fact more subtly in opposition to it, is sentimental pity, another aspect produced by TI/ME. So, here too one wants to remove a being's suffering, but for partly selfish (attached) reasons, hence not a wholistic motivation and one which will entrench the momentum of TI/ME.

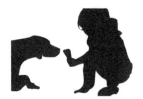

Figure 13.2: Felt-sense of compassion

13.4 *Mudita* (altruistic joy)

Mudita is a Pali word meaning joy, especially sympathetic or vicarious joy. It is the third pillar of the *brahmaviharas*. This is the pleasure that comes from delighting in other people's well-being. An example of this is the mind state and attitude of a parent observing a growing child's successes and accomplishments, or a friend's authentic happiness when you are promoted in your job.

Mudita can occasionally get confused with pride, yet a person feeling *mudita* may not have any interest or income from the accomplishments of the other. *Mudita* is, therefore, a pure joy unadulterated by self-interest and is actually a felt-sense appreciation of the subtle and essential connection you both share.

So, when we are happy in the joy other beings feel, it is called *mudita*; the opposite word is most aptly described by the Latin word *invidia*, meaning envy, a trait which is, conversely, encompassed by TI/ME.

◆ EXPERIENTIAL EXERCISE 19

Seeing beyond the I

◆ Sit comfortably in pairs facing each other.

◆ Keep your eyes gently closed for a minute or two.

◆ Open your eyes and look into the eyes of your partner for 10–20 minutes.

◆ Try not to blink too much (but blink if needed).

◆ Acknowledge the heart of your partner.

◆ Notice if you feel dazed, self-conscious, insecure, awkward and so on. Also, notice any vibrancy, enchantment, connection, absorption and so on.

◆ Are you wanting to avert your eyes? Or are they absorbing or being absorbed by your partner's eyes? If distracted, gently bring your gaze back.

◆ Let yourself be. Feel your emotions. Cry, laugh, moan, croak...

◆ Do you sense sadness or happiness in yourself and your partner?

◆ Provide relational space for each other.

◆ Realize any tension holding or passing inside you.

◆ Realize any closeness and gratitude arising.

◆ Is there anxiety in your core or is it peace?

◆ Can you feel the core of your partner?

◆ Talk with your partner about what you both felt during this exercise. There is often a lot to discuss.

◆ After this exercise you may notice how much easier it is to look into the eyes of another and how the gaze is very often met with a smile.

13.5 *Upekkha* (equanimity)

The real meaning of *upekkha* is equanimity, not indifference in the sense of being unconcerned for others. It is the fourth virtuous pillar of the *brahmaviharas*. When *upekkha* is considered as a spiritual virtue it means balance in the face of the vicissitudes of life. It is steadiness of mind, unshakeable fearlessness, a state of inner equipoise that cannot be upset by gain and loss, honour and dishonour, praise and blame, pleasure and pain. *Upekkha* is freedom from all points of self-reference; it is indifference only to the demands of the ego-self with its craving for pleasure and position, not to the well-being of one's fellow human beings. True equanimity is the crescendo of the four social virtues. It is last but certainly not least, and does not override or negate the preceding three. Actually, *upekkha* illuminates the other three in an anti-fragile way.

NB: Upekkha, and for that matter the rest of the *brahmaviharas*, is not to be mistaken for forgiveness. Forgiveness is, generally, an intention void of insight. This is because the person, people or even inanimate things cannot be truly met if they are not felt. If they are not felt, the impression of them being separate, in order to forgive them, will perpetuate the sense of self rather than dissipate it. Still, if forgiveness is the word you use to describe what has been outlined in this chapter, then a mere word doesn't really matter. It is the insight of the passing of TI/ME that fuels felt-sense and connection which is important.

13.6 *Tonglen*

Tonglen is the Tibetan term for giving and receiving. *Tong* means 'giving or sending' and *len* means 'receiving'. It is not one of the *brahmavihara* abodes per se, but it is a very worthy complementary practice. *Tonglen* is a Tibetan Buddhist practice whereby a person opens their awareness of calm intensity to include the suffering of another being. The sharing of this transformational felt-sense is claimed to lessen the other being's perception of being identified to thoughts and sensations (i.e. there is a reduction in their suffering).

13.7 Altruism

If you had the choice between hurting yourself or someone else in exchange for money, how altruistic do you think you'd be?

A study at the University of Oxford (UK) encouraged people to consider the dilemma of choosing between pain and profit.[2] It found that participants cared more about other people's well-being than their own. This study went against other research findings showing that people usually place their own needs and desires above those of others[3] – the premise behind believing in the selfishness[4] of most human beings.

The Oxford study was conducted by a psychology team,[5] which used pain and money as a way of investigating altruism. Everyone has their own pain threshold, so the first task was a pain calibration. Researchers administered electric shocks with electrodes attached to the wrists of 160 subjects, starting at an almost imperceptible level and increasing the intensity until the subject described the pain as intolerable. Individuals perceiving the discomfort of others on a computer screen were given the 'deciding' task of how many electric shocks were issued. The shocks they were in charge of came with rewards. The decider was in a position to choose between issuing, for example, seven shocks for ten pounds versus ten shocks for seven pounds, or seven shocks for ten pounds versus ten shocks for fifteen pounds.

Anyway, to cut a long story short, the study participants predictably did not like the pain of receiving a shock, because they were willing to make less money per shock on average to receive fewer of them. But people were willing to lose twice that amount per shock to hurt an anonymous other less![6]

The outcome of this study fits with a psychological effect coined by Crocker and colleagues as 'otherishness',[7] otherwise known as altruism.

May altruism continue to grow to be humanity's defining characteristic.

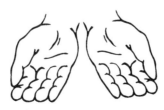

Figure 13.3: Sharing hands

Appendix 1: Process of Sensory Conditioning and Insight of TI/ME Passing

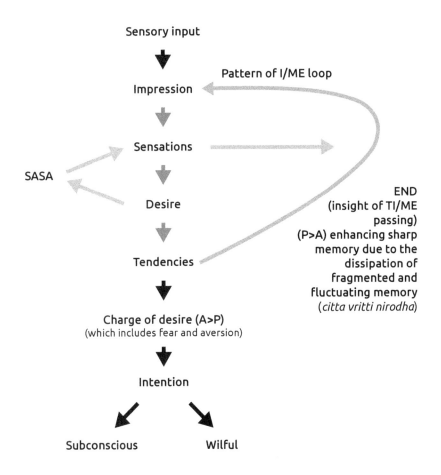

Sensory input

Impression

Pattern of I/ME loop

Sensations

SASA

Desire

Tendencies

END
(insight of TI/ME passing)
(P>A) enhancing sharp memory due to the dissipation of fragmented and fluctuating memory
(*citta vritti nirodha*)

Charge of desire (A>P)
(which includes fear and aversion)

Intention

Subconscious   Wilful

Appendix 2: Foundations for Feeling Safe and the Crescendo of Calm Intensity (Feeling HAPPI)

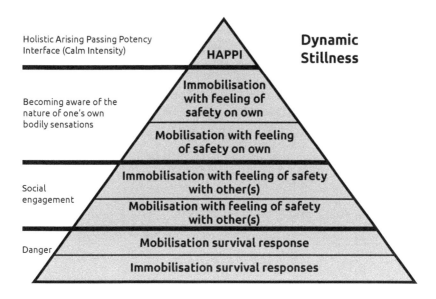

The diagram above illustrates that the survival responses are the base and prime objective of our autonomic nervous system to either immobilise in the face of extreme danger or mobilise in an escapable or defendable threat.

It goes on to show that when our body feels safe in the presence of another or others we can relax and rejuvenate by playing, chatting, sexually interrelating, meditating, etc. The diagram goes on to explain how the fluid-like safety of our system can be independently attained when there is a lessening reaction towards one's own sensations in addition to realizing their characteristic nature of arising and passing away.

The HAPPI aspect of the pyramid represents the crescendo of feeling safe like a wholistic fluid body of adaptable sensations, able to sense our original nature (dynamic stillness) both in oneself, and another. HAPPI is the subtle felt-sense awareness of equanimity which is an interface of insight between the relative (duality) and the absolute (non-duality).

Appendix 3: Meditation

Those bodywork therapists who have been in the field for a while have generally 'tuned up' enough for access attention to open the insightful presence of calm intensity. Nevertheless, it is important for the therapist to also understand that this is only opening to the subtler nature of being, it is not meditation (in the true sense of that word). Some bodywork therapists will naturally access a sense of wholeness without understanding it. These are usually the therapists who get beneficial results for their clients despite the past quantity of time spent acquiring skills, and consequently they often become quite popular as a therapist without trying. There can be an issue with this natural ability though, and that is a lack of understanding which can lead the therapist into believing that those times wholeness is not felt, and results are not achieved, are due to a client's blockages, or 'bad energy', rather than the therapist's own equanimity and insight being absent. As a result, these therapists either don't remain long in the bodywork field, or it is common for there to be a covert internal conflict which follows them through their practice. This is circumstance whereby meditation retreats are invaluable. However, it is not the only good reason to attend a meditation retreat, as will now be explained.

There is a danger which lurks in the minds of those who interpret non-duality as the negation of perceiving things dualistically. If an individual were to negate duality in his or her everyday life, she or he would concurrently ignore the distinctions and discriminations needed for practical living. Moreover, despite the perilous implications impacted by such a negating perspective, he or she would also start to distort and disregard the very meaning of the word meditation. This is because the individual would likely start to regard everything that they participated in as a kind of meditation. Thus, she or he would likely think it not necessary to undertake a meditation as a form of discipline/practice. This would be extremely unfortunate as deep subconscious doing (TI/ME) is very unlikely to surface enough for it to be perceived as passing without partaking in dedicated meditation practice (with right understanding). The real issue which comes about by negating duality is that meditation is considered a continual celebration of 'chilling out' rather than an inquiry into the depths of our own subconscious. And so superficial TI/ME is all that is ever noticed as passing, while deep TI/ME continues to cause subconscious reaction.

While life is indeed a celebration, from the point of view of the universe, it mostly gnaws with dis-satisfactoriness and suffering from the point of view of being an individual separate from the rest of the world. It is when one realizes that the latter perspective is a dominant theme, supported by TI/ME, that meditation practice is called for and has a potentially huge impact for our ability to help others, especially in the world of therapeutic bodywork.

In the therapeutic setting the presence of calm intensity provides the insight needed to help establish a relational field. This encourages and enhances the expression of health in another, but it is not meditation, at least not in the context I am attempting to impart (as will be explained below). Nevertheless, such presence motivates one to deepen into insight further and meditation practice is an invaluable tool to help enable this.

When you (the bodywork therapist) treat another person, with the awareness this book has been recommending, it is likely that your deeper patterns of TI/ME will come to the surface. For this reason, it is extremely useful to make space in your diary to attend a meditation retreat. Those retreats which cater for your comfort and safety, in addition to supporting you enough to allow these deep patterns to bubble up are ideal. It is good to have guidance with this endeavour, at least to start with and those meditation centres which provide guidance upon awareness of the arising and passing nature of sensations are undoubtedly the most useful.

Some bodywork practitioners might feel that it is not important to attend regular retreats, or that there are simply too many other priorities which need attending to in their life. Such practitioners may have become good at re-suppressing the deep patterns of TI/ME after they have surfaced from the depths. Yet, suppression of deep TI/ME, in this manner, serves benefit only for the short term (in order to attend to one's life in a balanced manner). After a while the re-suppression will start to feel like a cornflake stuck in the throat, which is unable to be swallowed fully and is unable to be spat out (metaphorically speaking). This is because once deep patterns of TI/ME surface they can never be completely supressed again. The potency, that was invested in keeping deep TI/ME supressed, will have been liberated somewhat. It is when the accrual of the 'cornflakes' build up to a point that is noticeable that joining a meditation retreat, if only to understand what meditation really is, can be a huge relief.

You may have noticed that I haven't used the word 'meditation' much throughout this book. This is because I consider this word to be somewhat sacred and I like to uphold its deeper meaning, as it is often used inappropriately, which then sacrifices both the potential and depth a bodyworker has to offer. Meditation, if combined with the word practice, and referred to in the context I am about to explain, is a practice which requires a number of important inclusions. Once meditation has been sufficiently understood and embodied, via such practice, then the activities of daily life can be partnered with mindfulness and, for the bodyworker especially, calm intensity. This will be clearly understood when one has fully appreciated the immense and somewhat paradoxical doing/non-doing nature of meditation practice. When insight and understanding are insufficient in this regard then the word meditation will be confused as merely being a form of superficial mind pacification.

It is way beyond the scope of this book to explain what meditation is, and any oversimplification is simply not it. The following details are, therefore, mentioned as a means to direct the reader to conducive places, which have the capacity to tangibly share what meditation is, and utilize any techniques which may be (and often are) necessary.

To help meditation practice and understanding establish in this way one must first find a conducive environment, preferably a retreat centre specifically set up for this purpose. It is especially useful when this place is relatively free from distractions.

It is ideal when there is a supportive team, those familiar with meditation practice, at hand to help with your endeavour. The team should be able to provide for your essential needs so you can meditate without too much disturbance. The team should also include a guiding teacher who is well-versed with the technical aspects involved with the practice and have good experience in helping guide the individual through any difficulties which might arise, especially when the deep TI/ME patterns surface.

A practice that promotes the abandonment of harmful habits is vital as a foundation, otherwise the mind simply cannot settle with the kind of attention necessary to access the subtle felt-sense (of TI/ME arising and passing).

The duration of foundational meditation training will be most beneficial if it is between a week and two weeks. Ten day Vipassana meditation retreats are ideal. A period less than this does not usually provide enough clock-time to access the felt-sense needed for insight to establish itself beyond being a mere experience. After this foundation period of meditation training, and one is back into the slipstream of worldly affairs, it is good for him or her to 'top-up' the 'insight-bank' for a dedicated period of time each day. This can be a game changer for the bodywork therapist as far as resourcing goes.

There is generally a minimal 'doing' component incorporated into meditation retreats such as the ones recommended at the end of this appendix. This 'doing' helps to prevent the mind from dissociating or getting bored, which can otherwise occur due to the extended duration of remaining still. This kind of doing also helps the felt-sense to reveal blind areas of the body-mind and unearth the 'sticky' TI/ME residing in its depths.

The volition and capacity to help others in society is enhanced by meditation and is also a factor which enables deeper meditation, and therefore deeper insight, particularly as a bodyworker practising engaged non-doing. The insight of TI/ME arising and passing is often radiating with non-doing presence in individuals who have recently completed a meditation retreat. This post-retreat period is a great opportunity for a bodyworker to witness how engaged non-doing beneficially affects others, which can sometimes be quite profound.

This brief overview of meditation practice fundamentals is mentioned here only to highlight the importance of undertaking real meditation. There are many reasons/benefits a bodyworker enters into meditation practice of this nature. The most important of which are to re-source one's capacity to help others and deepen one's insight into the passing of TI/ME. These two benefits help to support each other and are a boon for the experienced bodyworker.

So finally, this overview is to encourage the bodyworker to establish him or herself in the practice of meditation. A ten day meditation retreat is ideal in order to scientifically (without bias) explore the core crux of this book. It is actually the only real way to understand and 'make' sense (insightfully) of what has been mentioned. Especially if the content of this book has enticed you but you've been intellectually side-tracked trying to make sense of 'something' which needs experiencing in order to be understood.

A retreat at one of the many meditation centres, detailed on the www.dhamma.org website are ideal for meditation practice as explained in this appendix. Other internationally oriented websites such as the following might be useful too:

www.ashintejaniya.org
www.thebuddhistsociety.org
www.ubakhin-vipassana-meditation.org

Glossary

Pronunciation symbols and non-capitalization have been omitted.

Acr – Acronym
Chn = Chinese
Eng = English
Fr = French
Ger = German
Grk = Greek
Hw = Hawaiian
Jp = Japanese
Ltn = Latin
Pli = Pali
Sp = Spanish
Skt = Sanskrit
Tbn = Tibetian

AAA (Acr): Access, Attention, Anchor

Abbaya (Pli): Felt-sense of passing away

Abhidhamma (Pli); **Abhidharma** (Skt): Third century BCE and later Buddhist texts which contain detailed scholastic presentations of doctrinal material appearing in the Buddhist suttas. It also refers to the scholastic method itself as well as the field of knowledge that this method is said to study.

 The renowned Buddhist scholar, Bhikkhu Bodhi, called it an abstract and highly technical systemization of the Buddhist doctrine, which is simultaneously a philosophy and an ethics guide, all integrated into the framework of a programme for liberation from suffering.

Adhittana (Pli): Determination; resolve; discipline

Ad hominem (Ltn): Personal attack rather than reasoned argument

Ad infinitum (Ltn): To infinity and eternity

Advaita (Skt): Non-duality; not two; unity; highest truth

Agochari Mudra (Skt): Gazing at the tip of the nose while aware of sensations and/or levels of *kumbhaka*

Ahamkara (Skt): Self arrogating 'I'; ego; I am 'ness'; self consciousness; the base for Maya's power of projection. *Sattwic ahamkara:* egoism composed in the sense of goodness and virtue

Ai no muchi (Jp): Love-whip; paradox of stern affection 愛のムチ

Ajiva (Pli): Livelihood; way one conducts one's life

Ajjattham (Pli): Felt-sense of internality

Ajna (Skt): Third ventricle *akasha* (realized space)

Akasa (Pli): Realized space

Akasha (Skt): Realized space

Akkupa-Dhamma (Pli): Unshakeable; one who has attained full mastery over the absorptions

Anahata (Skt): Heart *chakra*; the vibration which regulates life from birth to death; unstruck beat – *nada* – sound

Anapana (Pli): Awareness on the touch of the natural uncontrolled breath. Focus at the end of the inner nostrils and space between the nose tip and upper lip (philtrum)

Anatta (Pli): No 'I'; felt-sense of no soul; beyond the idea of self

Anicca (Pli): Impermanence; ephemerality; change

ANS (Acr): Autonomic nervous system

Antara (Skt): Internal; within

Antarakasha (Skt): Inner space which forms the substratum of our own individual creation

Anti-fragile (Eng): Embodied equanimity; pliant adaptability to life's ups and downs

Appamanna (Pli): Boundless state

Appana (Pli): Absorption into object

A posteriori (Ltn): That following experience; empirical evidence

A priori (Ltn): That which comes before; knowing independent of experience

Asana (Skt): Posture; third limb of raja yoga

Asava (Pli): Canker; taint; mental intoxicant. Four types:
- *Kamasava* (sense desire)
- *Bhavasana* (desiring eternal existence)
- *Ditthasava* (holding on to (wrong) views)
- *Avijjasava* (ignorance)

Ashwinau (Skt): Divine power of earth; nose

Ashwini mudra (Skt): Mudra involving contraction and release of the anal sphincter muscle

Atama (Jp): Head; head feeling

Atendere (Ltn): Attention; to stretch or direct one's awareness towards an object of knowledge or experience

Atman (Skt): Higher self; supreme self

Atma Vichara (Skt): Self-inquiry; self-abidance; self-resting

Aturdido (Sp): Overwhelmed; not being able to think straight

Avidya (Skt): Ignorance; lack of wisdom; lack of insight; nescient

Avijja (Pli): Personality belief (*sakkaya-ditthi*); ignorance; lack of wisdom; lack of insight; nescient

Aufheben (Ger): Facing a problem and transcending it due to 'seeing through it'

Augenblick (Ger): The shortest of moments; 'the blink of an eye'

Ayama (Skt): Non-doing

Bahidda (Pli): Externally; felt-sense of externality

Bahidda va citte cittanupassi viharati (Pli): Observing the arising and passing nature of the thoughts in another

Bahidda va vedana vedananupassi viharati (Pli): Observing the arising and passing nature of the sensations in another

Bahir (Skt): External; outside

Bala (Pli): Powers:
- *Saddha* (faith)
- *Viriya* (energy)
- *Sati* (mindfulness)
- *Samadhi* (concentration)
- *Panna* (insight/wisdom)

Balayam (Skt): Rubbing of fingernails. Some say this stimulates hair growth

Beta beta (Jp): Feeling of stickiness

Bhanga (Pli): Dissolution of the gross perception of the body. If an individual is in the appropriate setting, such as a meditation retreat centre, such dissolution can open up the deeper insights to do with inherent dis-satisfactoriness and No I (*dukkha* and *anatta*). Obviously, this doesn't sound very appealing, and it can take some time before an individual realizes how important this kind of inquiry is (see Appendix 3). It is far beyond the scope of this book to elaborate on the desire to inquire into this (*visshudi*). But just to say that although the stage (it is not really a state) of body-mind dissolution can feel liberating, in the right setting, it will at some point unveil a fear of death (fear of No I) which is a subconscious fear deep within *everyone* other than those who have realized the reality of death and 'beyond' (*gotrabhu*). When one briefly touches upon the felt-sense of dissolution, but is not in a place conducive for meditation, there is often a craving for the feeling to stay, as it can seem very pleasurable. In such circumstance the feeling is unlikely to last very long as the lack of understanding of what it infers will result in the subtle sensations turning back into less subtle sensations the longer the 'pleasurable' state is identified with. Yet, in the right environment with the right resolve (*adhitthana*), support and guidance, unearthing the fear of No I (*anatta bhaya*), misery (*adinava*), deep aversion (*nibbedha*) and the overwhelming desire to be free from the craving for TI/ME continuing (*muccitu-kamyata*), will eventuate with the strong establishment of the most important ingredient in meditation practice – equanimity (*upekkha*). When equanimity is established sufficiently (*anuloma-citta*) then there can be an 'adaption-moment of consciousness' opening to a 'maturity-moment' (also referred to as entering the lineage – *gotrabhu-citta*).

Please refer to Appendix 3 for more practical advice regarding the above explanation.

One last note on this is that some people can get obsessed with these phases of meditation, to the point of being imprisoned by them. This is a point where Zen understanding can emancipate an individual from subtly trying to achieve a state/experience.

Bhava (Pli): Becoming; process of existence
- *Kamma bhava* (sensuous existence)
- *Rupa bhava* (fine-material existence)
- *Arupa bhava* (immaterial existence)

Bhaya (Pli): Fear; terror; frightfulness

Bhru (Skt): Eyebrow

Bhrumadya (Skt): Trigger point for ajna chakra

Bhu (Skt): Earth

Bhuchari mudra (Skt): Placing the thumb tip of one hand at the philtrum. With fingers together raising the little finger two centimetres and gazing at the nail. After three minutes, remove the hand and gaze at the impression formed. When the impression starts to dissolve, notice the process of dissolution. Once it has gone, notice the clarity of nothingness space it leaves behind. Also, notice the mind wanting to replace this space with something. Finally, notice the subtle body sensations resonating with the space.

Bio-nimbus (Eng): Aura; biosphere

Bodhichitta (Skt): Spontaneous wish to enter the gateless gate of non-duality, motivated by the compassion for all sentient beings. This is accompanied by the falling away of attachment to the illusion of an inherently existing self.

Boketto (Jp): Daydreaming; the act of gazing vacantly

Bori bori (Jp) ぼりぼり: Crunching sound

BP (Acr): Balance point

Brahma Muhurta (Skt): Period between 4am and 6am, deemed to be the most useful time to meditate

Brahma Nadi (Skt): Primal midline

Brahmavihara (Pli): Four sublime/divine abodes. Also known as four boundless states (*appamanna*).
- *Mettā* (loving kindness)
- *Karuṇā* (compassion)
- *Mudita* (altruistic joy)
- *Upekkha* (equanimity)

BS (Acr): Binary simplicity

Calm intensity (Eng): The felt-sense of whole body dissolution (*sampajanna*); this is a state catalyscd following the full body felt-sense awareness aspect of *sampajanna*, the sixth of the ten 'calm in-10-city' qualities

Cetana (Pli): Intention; volition. One of the seven mental factors (*cetasika*) inseparably bound up with conditioned consciousness. Others are:
- *Phassa* (mental impression)
- *Vedana* (feeling)
- *Sanna* (perception)
- *Samadhi* (concentration)
- *Jivita* (vitality)
- *Manasikara* (advertence)

Chakra (Skt): Wheel

Chatoyer (Fr): To shimmer with effervescence

Chiku chiku (Jp): Prickle-tingle sensation

Chikyu (Jp): Earth

Chitra Nadi (Skt): Subtle *nadi* in *shushumna* which lays dormant until *ida* and *pingala* are balanced

Chitta vritti (Skt): Mind patterns

Chong Mai (Chn): Primal midline

CI (Acr): Calm intensity. The culminating wholistic felt-sense of the body usually preceded by attention, the awareness of subtle sensations passing and a state of balanced awareness. It can be perceived as sense of fluid dissolution of the body ('mid-tide') or potency dissolution ('long-tide') or the whole body seeming to dissolve and yet be more present with minimal gross sensations. This is the phase of CITC which can lead to grey-zone intention if there is insufficient insight.

CITC (Acr): Calm in-10-city; the process of realizing calm intensity (CI); becoming a city dweller (aware of *purusha*)
1. **Attention** (SASA; stretching awareness)

2. **Passing and arising** (settling; felt-sense perception with increasing equanimity)
3. **Awareness and equanimity** (state of balanced awareness)
4. **Calm intensity** (wholistic perception; fluid dissolution ('mid-tide'); potency dissolution ('long-tide'))
5. **Insight** (felt-sense understanding of passing, no-thing, no-time, no-self)
6. **Dynamic stillness** (non-duality insight/felt-sense paradox)
7. **Primal midline/*Li*[1]** (self born from insight)
8. **Felt-sense connection** (insight of entanglement without misperception of being merged; engaged non-doing)
9. **Transmutation** (reorganization)
10. **Loving appreciation** (thought born from insight)

Cittass-ekaggata (Pli): One pointedness of the mind with a high degree of attention

Cogito ergo sum (Ltn): Dictum coined by philosopher René Descartes in 1637; 'I think, therefore I am'

CPG (Acr): Central pattern generator

Creatio ex nihilo (Ltn): Creation out of nothing

CSF (Acr): Cerebro spinal fluid

Cura te ipsum (Ltn): Take care of one's self; an exhortation to clinicians to deal with their own issues before addressing those of others

Daharakasha (Skt): Perceived space subtlety at the region of the gut *mool-adhara, swadhisthana, manipura*

Dara dara (Jp): Sensation or sound of sluggish, trickling fluid

De facto (Ltn): From the fact; distinguishing what's supposed to be from what is

Deva (Pli): Heavenly being; radiant one; deity; celestial being; invisible to the human eye

Dhamma (Pli): The true nature of a thing/phenomenon

Dharana (Skt): Establishing the mind at one point; practice of one pointedness

Dharma megha samadhi (Skt): The highest samadhi; the state of unclouded truth

Dhyana (Skt): Calm intensity awareness of arising and passing, when it is understood as an interface of both manifest and unmanifest, otherwise there will be no insight of TI/ME passing and *dhyana* in such a case is no more than a state of body dissociation. When *dhyana* is not present and understanding of being in touch with both manifest and unmanifest then it is merely a transcendental/absorption state of the mind without insight. Coming out of this state, one may feel resourced, but there is no insight of TI/ME passing and, therefore, the same reactive tendencies will dominate one's perception and being.

Dibba (Pli): Heavenly or divine:
- *Dibba-loka* (heavenly world, occupied by devas)
- *Dibba-cakkhu* (divine eye)
- *Dibba-sota* (divine ear)

Digdevata (Skt): Divine power of space; ears

Doki doki (Jp): Sound of heart when it's beating fast; sensation of excitement

Domanassa (Pli): Grief; mentally painful feeling. According to the *Adhidhamma*, grief is always associated to antipathy and grudge, and therefore is *karmically* unwholesome

Drishti (Skt): Seeing; gaze

DS (Acr): Dynamic stillness

Dukkha (Pli): Suffering; misery; dissatisfactoriness; the feeling that something is missing. Some traditions propose that Gautama the Buddha meant to differentiate *dukkha* from *domanassa* by confining one to bodily suffering and the other to mental/emotional suffering, respectively

Ekaggata (Pli): One pointedness; primary factor in all *jhanas*

Ekagrata (Skt): One pointedness

Enantiodromia (Grk): The tendency of things to change into their opposites, especially a supposed governing principle of natural cycles and of psychological development. A principle introduced to the west by the eminent psychiatrist Carl Jung

END (Acr): Engaged non-doing

Engi (Jp): Twelve-link chain of dependent origination

Epannoui (Fr): Blooming with radiant joy

ERV (Acr): Expiratory residual volume

Ex nihilo (Ltn): Out of nothing

Flaner (Fr): To stroll aimlessly; caught in a cycle of repetition

Fou Rire (Fr): Free laughter; crazy laugh; carefree laughter; fools laugh

Freudentranen (Ger): Tears of joy from a deep source

Fukouchu no saiwai (Jp): An unfortunate situation leading to a fortunate one

Gachi gachi (Jp): Stiff tension sensation like a rock

Geborgenheit (Ger): The feeling of returning home after being away for a long period of time; feeling of being intensely 'in the moment'

GOD (Acr): Gling of Dissolution or Gleam of Dissolution

Granthi (Skt): Psychic knot
- *Brahma* (sensual attachment)
- *Vishnu* (personal/emotional attachment)
- *Rudra* (*siddhi* attachment)

Grelotter (Fr): To shiver/tremor/shake

Guki (Jp): Twisting sensation with pain

Guna (Skt): Quality; characteristic. According to *sankhya* philosophy there are three constituent comic *gunas*:
- *Rajasic*
- *Sattvic*
- *Tamasic*

Gyurtog (Tbn): Change; everything changes

HAPPI (Acr): Holistic Arising Passing Potency Interface

Hara hara (Jp): Thrilling sensation

Hasta (Skt): Hand; tactility

Hikikomori (Jp): Hermit; recluse; withdrawn from society

Hiri hiri (Jp): Sore with subtle heat

Ho (Jp): Sensation of relief (e.g. relief of tension from the body)

Ho'oponopono (Hw): Practice of observing TI/ME in oneself to help others; literally translated into English as 'correction', or 'to make right'; using mantra-style affirmations to love, forgive oneself

Hridayakasha (Skt): Perceived space subtlety at the level of the heart; *Anahata chakra*

Ida (Skt): *Chandra Nadi*; running from *mooladhra* to *ajna*; controlling left side of the body

Ikigai (Jp): Reason for being; something to live for

Invidia (Ltn): Envy

Ipso facto (Ltn): The fact by itself

IRV (Acr): Inspiratory residual volume

Ishwara Pranidhana (Skt): Surrender to wholeness

Japa (Skt): Continuous repetition/rotation of mantra

Jara (Pli): Old age; demise

Jhana (Pli): Absorption into object. Eight 'levels' of absorption:
- *Vitakka, vicara, piti, sukha, ekaggata*
- *Piti, sukha, ekaggata*
- *Sukha, ekaggata*
- *Ekaggata*
- *Ekaggata, akasha*
- *Ekaggata, vinnana*
- *Ekaggata, sunnata*
- *Ekaggata*, neither *sanna* nor not *sanna*

Jnana (Skt): Knowledge; understanding

Joie de vivre (Fr): Exultation of spirit; cheerful joy of everything in life

Kalapa (Pli): Corporeal unit of existence constituting the beginning of insight of arising and passing

Kalpati (Skt): Imagination

Kama (Pli): Lust

Kama Sankappa (Pli): Lustful thought

Kamma (Pli): Action arising from wholesome or unwholesome volitions (*kusala* or *akusala-cetana*). Effect of intention

Kankaku (Jp): Sensation; feeling; intuition; impression

Kapalbhati (Skt): Cranial cleansing and mucus reducing technique

Kapalbhati pran-ayama (Skt): Exhalation-focused breathing technique used to raise the *tejas* and awareness of arising and passing, especially at *ajna chakra*

Kapalbhti (Skt): Phlegm cleansing technique of cranium using breath or water

Kara (Jp): Empty space

Karma (Skt): Action; effect of intention. Four types:
- *Sanchita* (stored; dense; thick)
- *Prarabhda* (cannot be retrieved)
- *Agami* (to be fructified)
- *Kriyamana* (effect of deeds in present life)

Karmendriya (Skt): Intention-based motor organs. Five physical organs of action:
- *Hasta*
- *Pada*
- *Vach*
- *Upastha*
- *Payu*

Kawa (Jp): River; skin

Kawaakari (Jp): The gleam of last light on a river's surface at dusk; the glow of a river in the darkness

Kaze (Jp): Wind

Kensho (Jp): From Zen tradition: *ken* means 'seeing', *sho* means 'nature, essence', Buddha-nature or dynamic stillness. Initial awakening

Kevala (Skt): Free from intention; whole; spontaneous; alone

Ki (Jp): Tree; energy

Koan (Jp); **Gong-an** (Chn); **Kong-an** (Korean); **Cong-an** (Viet-namese): A question posed by a master in the Zen (Chan) traditions, which cannot be answered by mere intellect or conceptualization. It can only be 'solved' by deep felt-sense intimacy with calm intensity and being able to share the insight of dynamic stillness.

Kokoro (Jp): Heart-mind

Kriya (Skt): Creative action leading to wholeness

Kumbhaka (Skt): Internal or external retention of breath

Kupamanduka (Skt): Literally means – frog in a well; the phrase is used in relation to a person who foolishly considers their knowledge horizon as the limit of all human knowledge (much like a frog imagines its well to be the largest water body and cannot imagine an ocean that might be far more immense)

Kuuki (Jp): Air; empty energy

Kuuki yomu (Jp) 空気読む: 'Reading air'; being aware of others and their needs

Laya (Skt): Dissolution; melting

Lex parsimoniae (Ltn): Law of succinctness; Occam's Razor; the simplest explanation is usually the correct one; the simplest is often hard to realize as thought gets in the way

Li (Ch): Organic patterns. Not the same meaning as the word *li* in the Confucian *ju* philosophy

Loka (Pli/Skt): Open space; realm of existence

Lokuttara (Pli): Beyond space and TI/ME (realms)

Maha Akasha (Skt): Wide perceptual field

Mahabhuta (Skt): The elements: space, air, fire, water and earth

Mahakala (Skt): Timelessness; destroyer of TI/ME

Mahi (Jp): Numb sensation

Majjhima patipada (Pli): Middle path; not getting attached to extremes; (Skt): *madhyama-pratipada*

Manipura chakra (Skt): Fire element of the coeliac ganglia

Mantra (Skt): Subtle vibration of sound

Mara (Pli): Personification of TI/ME

Marana (Pli): Passing of conditioned impression without awareness

Maya (Skt): Cause of the phenomenal world; illusion; magic show

Mettā (Pli): Loving kindness

Mimoso (Sp): Someone for whom affection involves touch

Modus operandi (Ltn): Method of operating

Mogu mogu (Jp): Combination of sound and movement of the mouth when eating

Momento mori (Ltn): Remember you will die

Momento vivre (Ltn): Remember to live

Mono no aware (Jp) もののあれ: The awareness of the impermanence of all things and the gentle sadness and wistfulness at their passing

Mori (Jp): Forest; tree vitality

Mu (Jp): Empty; no mind

Mudra (Skt): Gesture; presentation, sealing posture

Mumonkan (Jp) 無 関: Gateless barrier, or gateless gate

Murasaki (Jp) むるさき: Indigo; colour of the perception of the third ventricle prior to its transition to white light. In Japanese poetry, it denotes love and permanence

Murcha (Skt): Fainting; swooning; spiritual ignorance; delusion

Mushin (Jp) 無: No TI/ME

Muzu muzu (Jp): Uncomfortable feeling (often leg or genital area); restless leg feeling

Nada (Skt): Psychic, internal, cosmic sound

Nadi (Skt): Channel; meridian; current

Nama (Pli): Mind

Nanna (Pli): Understanding; knowledge

Nasikagra (Skt): Tip of nose

Neba neba (Jp): Sticky sensation

Nekkhamma (Pli): Renunciation; freedom from sensual lust

Nekokaburi (Jp): Feigned innocence (wolf in sheep's clothing)

Neti Neti (Skt): ('*Na-iti Na-iti*') No worldly experiences can explain samadhi. So, this literally means 'not this, not this'

Nibbana (Pli): Extinction of greed, hatred and delusion

Nimitta (Pli): Mental reflex image
  - *Parikamma* (preparatory image)
  - *Uggaha* (unsteady, unclear)
  - *Patibhaga* (entirely clear, ready to enable access concentration)

Nimitta (Skt): Instrumental cause

Nirodha (Pli): Extinction of *sankharas* (compare to Sanskrit translation)

Nirodha (Skt): Control of *vritti* (compare to Pali translation)

Nirvikalpa Samadhi (Skt): State in which the mind ceases to dominate and only pure consciousness remains, revealing itself to itself without objects of the mind hindering. Superconscious state where mental modifications cease to exist and there is a transcendence of the manifest world. Indeterminate perception.

Niyama (Skt): Personal discipline to render the mind tranquil

Non sequitur (Ltn): That which does not follow, from a logical perspective but not from an inherent perspective (e.g. a felt-sense perspective)

Noro noro (Jp): Slowly, but with torpidity rather than mindfulness

Nupassana (Pli): Contemplation

Ojas (Skt): Subtle fluids: especially noticed in sexual energy

Ojyama shimashita (Jp): When leaving someone's home the word used to acknowledge that you are grateful for them having you in their space

Ojyama shimasu (Jp): When entering someone's home the word used to indicate the awareness of disturbing their space, and gratitude for them accepting your presence

Oscitation (Eng): Yawning

Oto (Jp): Sound

Otsukaresama (Jp): Used to let someone know that you recognize their hard work and are thankful for it

Pada (Skt): Foot

Pancha Bhuta (Skt): Five elements of nature: earth, water, fire, air, ether (space)

Panna (Pli): Wisdom; insight

Paramatman (Skt): Absolute supreme self

Pariyatti (Pli): The wording of a doctrine

Passadhi (Pli): Tranquility

Paticcasamuppada (Pli): Twelve-link chain of dependent origination. It shows the conditionality and dependent nature of that uninterrupted flux of impressions, tendencies, memories and experience accumulated into what is conventionally called the ego or 'I'/'me' or separate self

- *Avijja* (ignorance)
- *Sankhara* (formations of TI/ME)
- *Vinnana* (conditioned consciousness)
- *Nama-rupa* (body and mind)
- *Salayatana* (six senses)
- *Phassa* (impression via sense contact)
- *Vedana* (feeling/sensations due to impression)
- *Tanha* (desiring to repeat or avoid sensation – reactive tendency leading to intention)
- *Upadana* (clinging to what is liked and dissociating from that which is disliked)
- *Bhava* (re-birth of conditioned reaction)

- *Jati* (law of nature resulting in the impressions showing their impermanence – ageing)
- *Marana* (passing of conditioned impression without awareness)

Patipatti (Pli): Practice; pursuance; distinguished from mere theoretical knowledge

Payu (Skt): Anus

Phassa (Pli): Impression via sense contact

Pingala (Skt): *Surya nadi*, running from *mooladhra* to *anja*: controlling right side of the body

Piri piri (Jp): Heat sensation on skin; burning on tongue like when tasting chilli; can be sensed as many very tiny tingling sensations when the heat has dissipated

Piti (Pli): Rapture/bliss

Plaisir (Fr): Pleasure

Poki poki (Jp): Cracking noise and sensation

Pradipa (Skt): Light, lantern, lightning, electricity

Prakriti (Skt): Individual nature; manifest and unmanifest nature (calm intensity); primordial matter. Qualities (*gunas*) consisting of *sattva, rajas, tamas*

Prana (Skt): Vital energy that functions in various ways for the preservation of the body and is closely associated with the mind

Pran-ayama (Skt): Techniques enabling control of the breath leading to the letting go of subconscious and conscious controlling of the breath

Pratyahara (Skt): Withdrawal and emancipation of the mind from the domination of the senses and sensual objects. When combined with *dharana* it enables a SOBA (state of balanced awareness), whereas calm intensity is *dhyana* when it is understood as an interface of both manifest and unmanifest, otherwise there will be no insight of TI/ME passing and *dhyana* in such a case is no more than a state of body dissociation. Fifth stage of raja yoga (Patanjali's eight limbs of yoga)

Pro bono (Ltn): For the good

Puraka (Skt): Filling up; inhalation

Purusha (Skt): Literally means 'Who dwells in the city'. In *sankhya* philosophy *purusha* designates pure consciousness, undefiled and unlimited by contact with *prakriti*

Qi (Chn): Energy

Rabu rabu (Jp): Romantic feeling

Raison d'être (Fr): The most important reason for someone's existence

Raja (Skt): Royal. Raja yoga is the union of duality and non-duality. The most authoritative text is Patanjali's yoga sutras. The nineteenth-century sage Vivekananda espoused this take on yoga.

Rajas (Skt): Active; restless; dynamism; egoic

Rasa (Skt): Tongue; taste

Ravir (Fr): Tantalize

Rddhi (Pli): Eight psychic powers:
- Replicate and project bodily image of oneself
- Make oneself invisible
- Pass through solid objects
- Sink into solid ground
- Walk on water
- Fly
- Touch the sun and moon with one's hand
- Ascend to the *loka* of *brahma*

REC (Acr): Ripples and eddy currents

Rechaka (Skt): Emptying; exhalation

Revelare (Ltn): Revelation; uncovering of an essential truth that was previously obscured or distorted

Rigpa (Tbn): A *dzogchen* term meaning 'flash of knowing the ground'; the knowing of original wakefulness

Rlung (Tbn): Wind energy

Rupa (Pli): Body form. One of the five groups of existence (*khandha*)

Saddha (Pli): Faith; unshakeable confidence; not blind faith

Sahita (Skt): Intentional; combined with; doing

Sakkaya-Ditthi (Pli): Personality belief; 20 kinds of personality belief. First five are the belief of the personality to be identical to:
- Corporeality
- Feeling
- Perception
- Mental formations
- Consciousness (based on the above)

Salayatana (Pli): The six sense bases of mental activity

Samadhi (Pli): One pointedness of awareness. Three stages:
- *Parikamma samadhi* (preparatory concentration)
- *Upacara samadhi* (neighbourhood concentration)
- *Appana samadhi* (attainment concentration)

Samadhi (Skt): State of unity with the object of meditation and universal consciousness. Observer, observation and observed are the same. Good not to confuse this with the Pali interpretation of *samadhi*, which is actually access attention (*prayahara/dharana*)

Samgimigyap (Tbn): Unfathomable by the mind; mind cannot capture; beyond the reach of the intellect

Samma (Pli): Balanced

Samma Samadhi (Pli): One pointedness of awareness with understanding of the three characteristics of existence (*anicca, dukkha, anatta*)

Samma Sankappa (Pli): Right thought

Sampajanna (Pli): Very important word to understand; the felt-sense clarity of consciousness; noticing the continuous passing away of experience at the subtlest level. In the Buddhist Pali *Suttas* this word is frequently combined with the word *sati* (awareness). It refers to the awareness and insight of arising/passing inherent in body sensations, sound, sight, smell, taste and the contents of the mind. With regard to body sensations, *sampajanna* insight can be at one isolated area of the body, or the whole body. I coined the term calm-intensity referring to the whole body felt-sense component of *sampajanna*. This whole body sense feels like the body is dissolving. However, this is only superficial compared to the total dissolution of bhanga (see bhanga), which leads to the insight of no-I (*anatta*).

Samsara (Pli & Skt): Round of rebirth; perpetual wandering; the sea of life ever restlessly heaving up and down, illustrating the continuous process of ever again being born, growing old, suffering and dying

Samskara (Skt): Formation of TI/ME; the roots of dissatisfactoriness (*vasanas* being the branches)

Samyama (Skt): *Dharana, dhyana* and *samadhi* – same. Observer, observation and observed – same

Sankalpa (Skt): Visualization, intention, imagination

Sankappa (Pli): Thought

Sankhara (Pli): Formation of TI/ME; the second link in the *paticcasamuppada*. One of the five groups of existence (*khandha*)

Sankhya (Skt): One of the six main systems of *Shaddarshana* (Indian philosophy). The philosophical basis of the yoga system

Sanna (Pli): Conditioned perception. One of the five groups of existence (*khandha*)

Sara Sara (Jp): Non-viscous feeling; like the synovial glide of a joint when moving

SASA (Acr): Specific Area of Sensation Awareness

Satchitananda (Skt): Existence/consciousness/bliss, which is an epithet and description for the subjective experience of the ultimate unchanging reality

Sati (Pli): Awareness; mindfulness

Satori (Jp): A pure experience in which the true nature of one's being is known directly. It is a temporary state that is experienced with increasing frequency and intensity

Sattva (Skt): Equilibrium; dynamic stillness; true essence; balance

Savikalpa (Skt): Determinate perception; analysis; formulation; fragmentation; distinction between subject and object; impressions

Sazanami (Jp): Gentle (subtle) wave sound

Shabda (Skt): Sound and object of the hearing sense and property of space

Shaki shaki (Jp): Moist crunchy crispness

Shambhavi (Skt): Name for Goddess Parvati. *Shambhavi mudra* is the gesture of gazing at *ajna*

Shikataganai (Jp) 仕 がない: It cannot be helped; accepting that some things are not of our control

Shiku shiku (Jp): Discrete sensation accompanied by crying

Shinrinyoko (Jp): Forest bathing

Shinzo (Jp): Heart organ

Shizen (Jp): Nature

Siddhi (Skt): Eight psychic powers
- *Anima* (subtlety)
- *Laghima* (lightness)
- *Prapti* (acquiring all)
- *Prakamya* (touching the most expansive)
- *Mahima* (increasing size at will)
- *Ishitvam* (control of arising and passing)
- *Vashitva* (control over everything)
- *Garima* (increasing weight at will)

Extra powers:
- *Avadhi* (clairvoyance)
- *Nada* (clairaudience)
- Telepathy

SOBA (Acr): State Of Balanced Awareness. This is equivalent to *pratyahara*, not *dhyana*

Sora (Jp): Sky

Sowa sowa (Jp): Fidgety; restless

Sparsha Tanmatra (Skt): The essence of the touch sense. Associated with *anahata chakra*

SPEND (Acr): Seeing Patterns with Engaged Non-Doing

Srishti (Skt): Creation

Sthairyam (Skt): Steadiness; balanced disposition

Sthira (Sthiti) (Skt): Still; steady, e.g. steadiness of the body or mind

Sui sui (Jp): Smooth feeling; no problem

Sukha (Pli): Happiness; rapture

Sunnata (Pli): Emptiness; nothingness

Sunyata (Skt): Emptiness; nothingness

Surya (Skt): Sun; vital prana; shine of the eyes

Sushumna (Skt): Fluid midline containing three more subtle midlines: *brahma*, *chitra* and *vajra nadi*

Suu suu (Jp): Sense of menthol/minty on skin or in body

Swadhisthana Chakra (Skt): Sacral water bed

Tamas (Skt): Inertia; darkness; ignorance; laziness; recalcitrance; lowest form of ego

Tanmatra (Skt): Subtle nature; quality or essence of the elements

Tan-tien (Chn): Access attention point below the navel

Tanto choku nyu (Jp) 単 直: Incisively getting to the point

Tantra (Skt): The word *tantra* has been commonly, but incorrectly, associated with solely sex-orientated union, given popular culture's salacious obsession with somatic and psychologic intimacy. *Tantra* has, therefore, been termed the 'yoga of ecstasy', motivated by nonsensical ritualistic lasciviousness. This is far from the diverse understanding of what tantra means to those Buddhist, Hindu and Jain practitioners who practise it.

Actually, *tantra* refers to the insight gleaned from 'touching' non-duality, in the world of relativity (i.e. duality). The intimate realization of duality really being non-duality.

It is by realizing the divine reality during one's own daily interactions. It is a simultaneous union of the feminine-masculine, yin-yang, and spirit-matter, and has the ultimate purpose of realizing the deep equipoise of non-duality.

So, it is the realization of life not being separate from death! Arising and passing.

Tapas (Skt): Working outside the habit; productive intensity; austerity

Te ('De') (Chn): Inner power; the virtue of non-virtuousness; moral character; inherent character; could be used in the same context as the Pali term *dhamma*

Teate (Jp) 当て: Putting or placing a hand. Also means treatment (*Te* = hand, *ate* = put or place)

Tejas (Skt): Heat; edge or tip of a flame

Tekipaki (Jp) テキパキ: Move fast and efficiently (opposite to *noro noro*)

TEND (Acr): Therapeutically Engaged Non-Doing

Thug-je (Tbn): Compassion; first part of the word refers to heart-mind

TI/ME (Acr): Tendency, Identification (and Impression), Memory, Expectation (and Experiential patterns)

Trataka (Skt): *Dharana* practice of steady gazing at one point to balance the mind

Tson-pa (Tbn): Diligence; commitment

Uday (Pli): Felt-sense of arising

Upacara (Pli): Access concentration

Upasamo (Pli): Peace

Upasthva (Skt): Genitals

Upekkha (Pli): Equanimity; balanced nature; non-reactivity

Uzuki (Jp): Subtle ache or twinge sensation

Vach (Skt): Voice

Vairagya (Skt): Detachment from the world and its cause; *vairagya* and *viveka* with awareness reveal the hidden *vasanas*

Vajra Nadi (Skt): *Nadi* based in the brain and flowing in *shushumna*: enables the flow of *ojas* and sexual energy

Varuna (Skt): Divine power of water; associated to tongue

Vasana (Skt): Tendency created in the mind by performing an action or by enjoyment, which then induces the person to repeat the action or to seek repletion of the enjoyment

Vayanupassana (Pli): Passing of sensations and TI/ME; fizzling away of the fetters

Vayu (Skt): Divine power of air; associated to skin

Vedana (Pli): Sensations. One of the five groups (aggregates) of existence

Vedanta (Skt): The last part of the sacred scriptures postulated to have been composed prior to 5000 BC. *Vedanta* teaches the ultimate aim and scope of these scriptures. It states that there is an end of conditioned knowledge, where there is a witnessing of the mind's limits, a perception which realizes that which the conventional senses cannot perceive. It upholds the doctrine of either non-dualism (*advaita Vedanta*) or conditional non-dualism (*vishishta Advaita*)

Vicara (Pli): Sustained thought; sustained conception

Vidya (Skt): 'From the root'; inner knowledge

Vihara (Pli): Spiritual and psychological abodes; three abodes:
- Heavenly (*dibba-vihara*)
- Divine (*brahma-vihara*)
- Noble (*ariya-vihara*)

Vijja (Pli): Insight; higher knowledge; gnosis

Vikalpa (Skt): According to Patanjali, *vikalpa* is one of five types of thought, being fantasy/imagination. (The four other types of thought are right knowledge, misapprehension, deep sleep and memory.)

Vinnana (Pli): Consciousness. One of the five groups of existence (*khandha*)

Vinnana-Sota (Pli): Stream of consciousness

Vinyasa (Skt): To move in a special way; to move with intention; linking A to B with breath; breath-synchronized movement

Vipassana (Pli): Insight of nature as it is

Vishishta (Skt): Distinguished; distinct; particular; special; peculiar

Vishuddha (Skt): Throat chakra; purification centre

Vitakka (Pli): Thought; conception

Viveka (Skt): Discriminating discernment

Vivre membre leti (Ltn): Live remembering death

Vritti (Skt): Patterns arising in consciousness, like the eddy currents of a running stream

Vyoma Panchaka (Skt): Five subtle spaces within consciousness:
- *Guna rahita akasha*
- *Param akasha*
- *Maha akasha*
- *Tattwa akasha*
- *Surya akasha*

Wa (Jp) 和: Harmony; importance of avoiding conflict to maintain a state of balance

Wabi-sabi (Jp): A way of living that focuses on finding beauty within the imperfections of life and peacefully accepting the natural cycle of life, especially the passing away of phenomena

Waku waku (Jp): Collective feeling of excitement

Wanderlust (Ger): The desire to explore and not stay caught in a habit

Waza waza (Jp): Wilful intention

Wei wu wei (Chn): The action of non-doing

WOSI (Acr): Weight, Outline, Skin, Internal sense

WOW (Acr): Wing Opening Awareness

Wu ge yaosu (Chn): Five elements of nature: earth, water, metal, fire, air

Wu ji (Chn): Great primordial emptiness

Wumenguan (Chn): Gateless barrier. A collection of 48 Chan koans compiled in the early thirteenth century by the Chan master Wumen Huikai 1183–1260 (Mumon Ekai)

Wu wei 無爲 (Chn/Pin-Yin): By non-doing everything is done. END therapist interpretation: by not reacting to TI/ME, health gets to express itself. *Wu wei* is the 'practice' of realizing the *Tao* and *Tao* is the essence of *Wu wei*.

Wu wei (Chn, Pin-Yin), *li* (Chn, Pin-Yin), *wabi-sabi* (Jp), *dhamma* (Pli), *laya* (Skt) all complement one another in helping to perceive and understand the felt-sense of nature. It is also relevant to translate this in the therapeutic setting into: 'By seeking nothing, everything is found'.

Yama (Skt): Doing; Self-restraints which render the emotions tranquil

Yatha bhuta (Pli): The expression of reality as it is, rather than any preference one might have

Zeitgeist (Ger): The prevalent spirit or mood of an era, as shown by ideas and beliefs of the time

Zhun (Chn): Love for humanity (Confucian term)

Ziran/Tzu Jan (Chn): Naturally so, of itself. The condition that something will be in if it is permitted to exist and develop naturally and without interference or conflict

Zoku zoku (Jp): Sensation of tingling up the spine

Zuki zuki (Jp): The feeling of a subtle throbbing agitation

Zukin zukin (Jp): The feeling of severe gross throbbing

References

Austin, J.H. (1999) *ZEN and the BRAIN*. London: MIT Press.

Bohannon, J. (2014) 'Electric shock study suggests we'd rather hurt ourselves than others.' www.sciencemag.org.

Calais-Germain, B. (2006) *Anatomy of Breathing*. Seattle, WA: Eastern Press.

Cassidy, J. and Shaver, P.R. (1999) *Handbook of Attachment. Theory, Research, and Clinical Application*. New York, NY: Guilford Press.

Clarke, B. (2011) *Yin Yoga. The Philosophy & Practice of Yin Yoga*. Vancouver, Canada: Wild Strawberry Productions.

Crocker, J., Canevello, A. and Brown, A. (2016) 'Social motivation costs and benefits of selfishness and otherishness.' *Annual Review of Psychology*, 68: 299–325.

Crockett, M.J., Kurth-Nelson, Z., Siegle, J.Z., Dayan, P. and Dolan, R.J. (2014) 'Harm to others outweighs harm to self in moral decision making.' *Proceedings of the National Academy of Sciences*, 111(48) 17320–17325.

Dispenza, J. (2014) *You are the Placebo: Making Your Mind Matter*. Sydney: Hay House.

Dispenza, J. (2017) *Becoming Supernatural*. London: Hay House.

Flavell, J. (1979) 'Metacognition and cognitive monitoring: A new area of cognitive developmental inquiry.' *American Psychologist*, 34(10) 906.

Frydman, M. and Dikshit, S.S. (2008) *I Am That. Talks with Sri Nisar-gadatta Maharaj*. Durham, NC: The Acorn Press.

Gilder, L. (2009) *The Age of Entanglement: When Quantum Physics Was Reborn*. New York, NY: Vintage Publications.

Gregory, J. (2018) *Effortless Living*. Rochester, VT: Inner Traditions/Bear.

Harris, A. (2019) *Conscious: A Brief Guide to the Fundamental Mystery of the Mind*. New York, NY: HarperCollins.

Kaiser, F., Coudreau, T., Milman, P. and Ostrowsky, D.B. (2012) 'Entanglement-enabled delayed choice experiment.' *Science*, 338(6107) 637–640.

Kotler, S. (2015) *The Rise of Superman. Decoding the Science of Ultimate Human Performance*. London: Quercus Books.

Krishnamurti, J. and Bohm, D. (1985) *The Ending of Time*. San Francisco, CA: HarperCollins.

Laughlin, K. (2014) *Stretching & Flexibility*. Sydney: Body Press.

Laughlin, K. (2016) *Overcome Neck & Back Pain, 4th Edition*. NSW: BodyPress.

LeBlanc, J., Dulak, S., Cote, J. and Girad, B. (1975) 'Autonomic nervous system and adaptation to cold in man.' *Journal of Applied Physiology*, 39(2) 181–186.

Maté, G. (2009) *In the Realm of Hungry Ghosts*. London: Random House.

McGilchrist, I. (2009) *The Master and His Emissary*. New Haven, CT: Yale University Press.

McKeown, P. (2015) *The Oxygen Advantage*. New York, NY: William Morrow Publishing.

Miller, D.T. (1999) 'The norm of self interest.' *American Psychology*, 54: 1053–1060.

Mott, M. (2005) 'Did animals sense tsunami was coming?' *National Geographic*. Available at https://www.nationalgeographic.com/animals/article/news-animals-tsunami-sense-coming.

Peruzzo, A., Shadbolt, P., Brunne, N., Popescu, S. and O'Brien, J.L. (2012) 'A quantum delayed-choice experiment.' *Science*, 338(6107) 634–637.

Piff, P.K., Stancato, D.M., Cote, S., Mendoza-Denton, R. and Keltner, D. (2012) 'Higher social class predicts increased unethical behaviour.' *Proceedings of the National Academy of Sciences*, 109(11) 4086–4091.

Pike, A. (2008) 'Bodymindfulness in physiotherapy for the management of long standing chronic pain.' *Physical Therapy Reviews*, 13(1) 45–56.

Porges, S. (2004) 'Neuroception, a subconscious system for detecting threats and safety.' *Zero to Three*, 24(5) 19–24.

Porges, S. (2011) 'The polyvagal theory: New insight into adaptive reactions of the autonomic nervous system.' *Cleveland Clinic Journal of Medicine*, 76(2) S86–S90.

Ramachandran, V.S. (2012) *The Tell-Tale Brain. A Neuroscientist's Quest for What Makes Us Human*. New York, NY: W.W. Norton.

Rosenberg, S. (2018) *The Healing Power of the Vagus Nerve: Self-Help Exercises for Anxiety, Depression, Trauma and Autism*. Berkeley, CA: North Atlantic Books.

Rothschild, B. (2000) *The Body Remembers. The Psychophysiology of Trauma and Trauma Treatment*. New York, NY: W.W. Norton.

Rovelli, C. (2016) *Seven Brief Lessons on Physics*. London: Penguin, Random House.

Schore, A.N. (1994) *Affect Regulation and the Origin of the Self*. Hillsdale, NJ: Lawrence Erlbaum Associates.

Spira, R. (2017) *Being Aware of Being Aware*. Oxford: Sahaja Publications.

Spira, R. (2021) *A meditation on; I am*. Sahaja Publications: Oakland, CA.

Stevenson, D. (2002) *Hoofprint of the Ox: Principles of the Chan Buddhist Path as Taught by a Modern Chinese Master (Master Sheng-yen)*. Oxford: Oxford University Press.

Sumner, G. and Haines, S. (2010) *Cranial Intelligence*. London: Singing Dragon.

Taleb, N. (2013) *Antifragile*. London: Penguin Books.

Walker, P. (2015) *The Tao of Fully Feeling. Harvesting Forgiveness out of Blame*. Lafayette, CA: Azure Coyote Publishing.

Wallace, B.A. (2010) *Distorted Visions of Buddhism: Agnostic and Atheist*. New York, NY: Spiegel & Grau.

Wilson, T. *et al.* (2014) 'Just think: The challenges of the dis-engaged mind.' *Science*, 345(6192) 75–77.

Endnotes

Preface

1   Here 'E' stands for expectations (future), and also for experience (past), but not experiencing (which is present).
2   Tendencies, Impressions, Memory fluctuations, Expectations.

Chapter 1

1   It's useful to remember that many people don't even manage to apply enough focused attention to perceive the black dot for long enough to be aware of its qualities, let alone the white paper.
2   A term coined by the German philosopher, Immanuel Kant. Noumena describes the thing which is independent of human sense perception. However, as soon as the mind interprets and isolates the felt-sense of wholeness into a 'thing', then insight is clouded by TI/ME. Therefore, any philosophy, be it from a materialist or idealist/ metaphysical perspective, may promote the known, but in the same moment it will prevent 'knowing'.
3   The movie analogy was inspired by Professor David Bohm who often used it in his talks on consciousness. Also, an analogy often used by Rupert Spira.
4   A premise which most, if not all, philosophies seem to struggle with.

Chapter 2

1   From the Latin *salvare* meaning salvation.
2   The 'anomaly detector' is the term used by Professor Vilayanur Ramachandran to describe the nervous system being stuck in 'on mode'. See: *The Tell-Tale Brain* (2012), by V.S. Ramachandran. New York, NY: W.W. Norton.
3   See: Taleb, N. (2013) *Antifragile*. London: Penguin Books.
4   This fits with the Hegelian philosophy of *Aufheben*.
5   See: Cassidy, J. and Shaver, P.R. (1999) *Handbook of Attachment: Theory, Research, and Clinical Application*. New York, NY: Guilford Press..
6   See: LeBlanc, J. *et al.* (1975) 'Autonomic nervous system and adaptation to cold in man.' *Journal of Applied Physiology,* 39(2) 181–186.
7   Or: embodied non-doing.
8   See Rothschild, B. (2000) *The Body Remembers: The Psychophysiology of Trauma and Trauma Treatment*. New York, NY: W.W. Norton & Company.
9   So, the ANS basically ends up responding to what is either perceived as a threat or what feels safe. Interestingly, the perceptual input with most adult humans is approximately 80 per cent from memory and only 20 per cent from the senses picking up

environmental information. This is because by the time we are a conditioned adult the majority of information processed by the ANS is a combination of impressions left by a past experience, or expectations projected on top of input fed by the senses. That means our brain-stem driven behaviour is mostly not responding to a present reality, we are in fact mostly reacting to the past and/or the future.

Here's a hypothetical scenario to muse over. If the perception of an individual were almost entirely influenced by memory and/or projection but hardly at all by the 'in-touch' senses, then the person would be considered either asleep or somewhat dissociated. Whereas, if the individual's perception was mostly influenced by the here and now senses, rather than memories and/or projections, then the person would be operating presently, yet primitively, as perception would not have much reference fed from past events or possible futures. But consider this, when a person perceives the environment as being safe, and there is a learned ability to feed the ANS with equal amounts of sensory and conditioned input, then the person's physiology becomes present in a very wholistic way – it tingles with aliveness. The body wakes up to itself and responds to circumstance in an embodied rather than distorted manner.

Intriguingly, if the ANS is 'trained' to be more aware of real time sensory input and adapt to the input rather than react to it, then one's physiology is no longer at the mercy of narrative-fed impressions from the past, or expectations of an imagined future, while still being able to orient to these aspects of psychologic time when necessary.

When a therapist is embodied in this way they can help a client to also adapt their perception of experience by acting as a non-reactive reference. A therapist who adapts to experience without reaction will enhance physiologic co-regulation with a client's ANS and help it to continue learning, functioning and relating with the world in a present manner.

On the other hand, when a therapist's perception is caught in reactive tendencies, fuelled by the past and future, then the client's mind is not able to distinguish real-time sensory input from past impressions and so the felt-sense of their body will be more vulnerable to continue this cycle by all manner of different behaviour patterns leading to different forms of intermittent dissociation and feeling dis-regulated.

Dissociation of this kind is a survival response which needs to be met with a perception that has the capacity to help integrate, and that requires integration in the therapist first.

Continuous subconscious reactions taking place in our stimulating and impactful world will very often lead to overwhelm, whether we realize it or not. The therapist is there to help a client gather themselves together and gradually perceive more wholeness by helping her or him soften into the flow of safety. Yet, by far the most valuable contribution a therapist provides is by encouraging the fluid nature of the client to be touched with the felt-sense insight of their own inherent anti-fragility. In other words, the therapist helps the client claim the insight of their original nature by being in felt-sense contact with original nature.

Therefore, a specific environment with relevant sensory input, can serve as a reference for safety when an individual's system becomes overwhelmed. However, if this reference becomes relied upon, and the client doesn't discover their own inherent resource, then fluid-like safety will be limited, due to dependence on a specific environment, contact and sensory input. So, an END therapist empowers a client to embody an anti-fragile disposition. This enables the individual to reduce their reactive fear/desire, which was based upon a prior encounter/stimulus.

10   This can be likened to secure attachment (from the child development literature). However, this runs even deeper as insight of TI/ME passing (see endnote 23) will also help attachment to another dissipate, until the stream of inquiry doesn't need another to return to for security. This of course is likely to happen, in the end,

following the development of a child's healthy secure attachment, but insight will likely not be encouraged, as society's main thrust is for honouring the intentional accumulation of TI/ME.

11 Safe by being empowered to sense that there is no need to react with protection and embodying how this feels. This results in promoting the ability to accommodate, feel and adapt to future relational interactions.

12 Autonomic nervous system imbalance seems to be the root cause for most pathologies which humans encounter. It is not just END therapists who share this perspective.

13 Neuroception is a term coined by Stephen Porges to describe whether situations and/or people are dangerous, or life threatening. Porges, S. (2004) 'Neuroception, a subconscious system for detecting threats and safety.' *Zero to Three,* 24(5) 19–24.

14 With others and the environment in general.

15 The majority of clients will not realize this, but they will react to it regardless of their being conscious of it or not.

16 Original health is non-dualistic, therefore it is neither not-health or its opposite.

17 Original nature is what Jiddu Krishnamurti called the 'vibrant ground beyond emptiness' as he attempted to share its nature as both the source of stillness, and the essence of a divisionless movement (vibration).

18 This is not a form of 'neurophilosophy' (as mentioned in Iain McGlichrist's (2009) book *The Master and His Emissary.* New Haven, CT: Yale University Press.) as it is unlikely for philosophy, of any kind, to get beyond its own terms of reference and its own epistemology.

19 Dispenza, J. (2017) *Becoming Supernatural.* London: Hay House.

20 Health here is in the context of a biodynamic non-dual perspective, which has no opposite.

21 All concepts are born from a dualistic perspective.

22 Jiddu Krishnamurti was a famous twentieth-century spiritual teacher who was able to articulate non-duality in a way very few have done before him, or since.

23 See Krishnamurti, J. and Bohm, D. (1985) *The Ending of Time.* San Francisco, CA: HarperCollins.

24 The acronym TI/ME, standing for tendencies, impressions (and identification), memory formulation/fluctuation, and expectations, will be used frequently through this book to stand for psychologic time and the undercurrent of intention. The ancient Chinese referred to TI/ME as the 'ten thousand things'. A larger number is not used as there was no word for a larger number in that period – if there was it would have been used instead.

25 Even those words wishing to describe connection. This is because such words imply that there is originally a state of separation.

26 Verbs are more intimate with non-duality than nouns.

27 For a very useful talk by Rupert Spira on the use of words relating to non-duality, and the benefit of not being fixated by them, check out this YouTube link: www.youtube.com/watch?v=0hsb8Xxt1M0.

28 Stretching of awareness is attention. A term Rupert Spira often uses in his talks.

29 A *koan* is a paradoxical anecdote or riddle which has no solution other than by realizing the limitation of thought.

30 The *ch'an* tradition includes specific meditation practice deriving from dhyana (concentration) meditation principles found in the orthodox teachings of Gautama the Buddha.

31 In Japanese this is called *mumonkan*: the 'gateless gate'.

32 Through awareness of the delusion (mask) we base ourselves on there is a dissipation of the tendencies that the delusion is founded on. So there is not actually an intent to discard. The term discarded just means that the delusion is seen for what it is and cannot continue to exist as a delusion.

33 When the quality of this arising and passing is perceived as non-dual then the delusion of separation and objects dissolves to leave insight in its wake, i.e. A = P (arising is the same as passing), much the same way that $E = MC^2$ (energy is the same as mass times the speed of light squared). It is interesting to note that the Welsh mathematician, Robert Recorde, first used the two lines of the equals sign to denote two seemingly different lines of exactly the same length. These lines correspond to the equivalent of a 'wormhole'/tunnel connecting one side to the other and revealing the two sides as the same despite another angle of perception seeing them as different.

34 This is an example often used by Rupert Spira during the meetings he conducts. Used here with permission. Spira, R. (2017) *Being Aware of Being Aware.* Oxford: Sahaja Publications.

35 Term for a perceivable aura surrounding a biologic entity.

Chapter 3

1 Most people are just not comfortable in their own heads, according to a new psychological investigation led by the University of Virginia. The investigation found that most would rather be doing something – possibly even hurting themselves – than doing nothing or sitting alone with their thoughts. Timothy Wilson and colleagues conducted a series of 11 studies at the University of Virginia and Harvard University, finding that participants from a range of ages generally did not enjoy spending even brief periods of time alone in a room with nothing to do but think, ponder or daydream. The participants, by and large, enjoyed much more external activities such as using a smartphone or listening to music. Some actually preferred to give themselves mild electric shocks than to be in a situation of non-doing! See: Wilson, T. *et al.* (2014) 'Just think: The challenges of the dis-engaged mind.' *Science,* 345(6192) 75–77.

2 Apart from 'intentional attention'. Q: What prevents us being aware of the screen of our original nature? A: Intent born from TI/ME.

3 Gross sensations can be anything like pressure, heaviness, pain, tightness, tension, contraction, buzzing and so on. Subtle sensations can be hard to label, but they can be tingling, trickling, flowing, expanding and so on.

4 The aspect of 'effort' in effortless effort.

5 Which includes especially thought.

6 Content of thought: the main aspects being TIIIIMEE (tendencies, impressions, identification, interpretations, intention, memories, expectations, experiences). There is a lot of 'I' in TI/ME.

7 Such exposure, with understanding, is the basis of insight.

8 J. Krishnamurti often emphasized the importance of the 'act' of non-doing in relationship.

9 Intention being a core pillar of the contents of thought without insight (I, me, mine).

10 The felt-sense of sensations arising and passing. In the ancient Indian language of Pali, this is called uday-abbaya-nupassana. The awareness of passing is the most important. This is called vayanupassana.

11 It is only considered paradox from a dualistic either/or perspective.

12 Rovelli, C. (2016) *Seven Brief Lessons on Physics.* London: Penguin, Random House.

13 TI/ME – the hidden 'I' and 'ME' of TIME.

14 Intention can be both conscious and subconscious in this regard. This is because subconscious reactions to sensory input include thoughts, experiences, memories and so on, which are based on the impression of being a separate individual. This is the same premise that guides conscious responses to sensory input.

15 The more we practise this kind of conscious attention, the more awareness will replace such intention with natural/relational non-reactivity.

16 Health in this context is how we perceive it as biodynamic craniosacral therapists, i.e. the expression of intelligence which does not have an opposite. We could talk about health and the differing levels and varying degrees of it, yet as soon as we entertain the words 'differing' and 'varying' we surreptitiously invite less and more, which cloud the essence of what we are considering health here (the word cloud here implies duality and thought requiring opposites to elucidate meaning).

17 Intention prevents stillness and its natural effect on releasing tension held within the tissues (in-tension). Q: What is holding the tissues in the first place? A: Intention. What a viscous cycle! Q: Why does intention have this effect? A: Because intention (to do this or that) doesn't allow the vital space for the organizing intelligence of the body to unfold into its natural inherent stillness.

18 Pleasure/pain; good/bad; right/wrong; positive/negative and so on are all evaluative perceptions. It is the tendency of like and dislike that provides the reactive charge for desire and intention.

19 Keep returning to Appendix 1 throughout this book. It contains an orientating map and an important link for establishing non-doing.

20 We are not merely machines. It just takes a period to settle the mind, with clear awareness of our subtlest sensations, to realize this. 'Consciousness' is the word we interpret through apperception. Yet the reality, beyond apperception and that which the word distorts, is what is perceived despite the senses and the accumulation of the past. Check it out – one might call this approach first-hand science. Rupert Spira goes into great depth and detail on this matter in his book: *Being Aware of Being Aware* (2017) Oxford: Sahaja Publications.

21 Pike, A. (2008) 'Bodymindfulness in physiotherapy for the management of long-standing chronic pain.' *Physical Therapy Reviews*, 13(1) 45–56.

22 Resulting in subconscious motor intention.

23 Insight in this context is not association, it is the felt-sense realization of sensations arising and passing within ourselves and the client.

24 Mind *is* movement.

25 A short tale written by Danish author Hans Christian Andersen about two weavers who promise an emperor a new suit of clothes that they say is invisible to those who are unfit for their positions, stupid or incompetent – while in reality, they make no clothes at all, making everyone believe the clothes are invisible to them. When the emperor parades before his subjects in his new 'clothes', no one dares to say that they do not see any suit of clothes on him for fear that they will be seen as stupid. Finally a child cries out, 'But he isn't wearing anything at all!'

26 Without insight of change the expression of health will never be optimal.

27 That being said, if the sense of a tide arises, free from such intent, then this calm/deepening movement of the mind enhances the potential for insightful stillness to reveal itself, which is useful for encouraging the expression of health (an understatement if ever there was one!).

28 Spurious impression, understanding and projection of tides and midlines.

29 Releasing it happens just by being aware of it and not trying to change it.

30 See: Stevenson, D. (2002) *Hoofprint of the Ox: Principles of the Chan Buddhist Path as Taught by a Modern Chinese Master (Master Sheng-yen)*. Oxford: Oxford University Press.

31 Mind here is the same as TI/ME.

32 'No mind' is not to be mistaken for being mindless.

33 Not reacting to pleasant sensations is so hard because the tendency of the mind is primed to want more pleasure and for pleasure to cover over the unpleasant (sensations or memory; experience being both). Pleasant sensations do not last despite memory trying to sustain and reignite them. Just the same way that unpleasant sensations do not last if we let go of the resistance towards them. All sensations are changing by nature, just as the mind is moving by nature. The witnessing of this fact

is neither changing or moving (based on division), yet it is the essence of divisionless movement.

34 J. Krishnamurti and David Bohm used to have dialogues which would reach a point where they would be talking about the 'ground'. They were using this word as they both agreed that this was the most appropriate term to try and describe the source of our being. In biodynamic craniosacral therapy circles it is known as dynamic stillness.

35 Sensation and impression are only separated due to conceptualization, the same way that body and mind are separated by concept.

36 Access attention acts as a platform for inquiry and opening to the insight of the felt-sense, i.e. arising and passing.

37 *Attendere*: Latin verb which translates to awaiting while stretching one's awareness.

38 It could be metaphorically likened to the National Aeronautics and Space Administration (NASA) in the USA in the way it helps to launch attention to enter the stratosphere of awareness and insight.

39 Which is insight of the passing nature of TI/ME – reactive Tendencies, Impressions (such as images in the mind), fluctuating Memory formulation/fluctuation (past) and Expectation (future).

40 Some people can struggle, or get zoned out, with some of the more subtle access areas, especially those involving sound or light. The 'tone' and 'shine' of consciousness require a disposition of considerable attentiveness. For example, the attentive awareness of the exquisitely subtle high pitched sound of the central nervous system. This does not suit some people and so the specific areas of sensation awareness, such as breath touching the groove of the philtrum, are sufficient to access the insight of arising and passing.

41 This is not an intention to 'drop' intention, as this will form a cycle of doing based on intention.

42 The party being the relational field.

43 Cupid's bow is the name given to the delineating curve formed between the valley-like groove of the philtrum and the mid-body of the upper lip.

Chapter 4

1 Reactive Tendencies, Impressions (such as images in the mind) and/or Intention and/or Identification, Memory fluctuation (explicit), Expectation and/or fragmented body sensation-based experience (implicit).

2 Tendency to identify and react to an event, object, interaction and so on by liking or disliking, wanting or not wanting, desire or aversion.

3 The 'I' of TIME can also stand for identification.

4 Memory fluctuation and instability. Citta vritti. Past.

5 Projections. Future.

6 Be warned, the acronym TI/ME will be mentioned multiple times throughout this book and if not understood will likely become somewhat nauseating.

7 Potency is the term used by biodynamic craniosacral therapists to describe the felt-sense of subtle health expression. Perceived with insight, it is the felt-sense awareness of TI/ME passing – and the fresh arising/passing vibration free from TIME.

8 Mind is movement, regardless of how still it may appear. One can explore this by looking at a mobile phone screen. Look at it for a minute or two, then close the eyes and pay attention to the motion of light in the region of the 'third eye'. Notice how the light impressions are all fragmented to begin with. When the mind settles, a rhythm unfolds, which might also be felt through the body. As this movement throughout the body slows down it might feel like a nurturing flow free from intention. However, it is still the motion of the doing mind, albeit much more subtle than usual. When

there is an observer separate from the observed, then there is duality – this is not non-doing.

9   As a therapist it is good NOT to translate the potency of presence as something we 'surf' on, or with. When our midline resonates and witnesses the potency of another, it doesn't play, manipulate or get carried away by it, despite the mind's subtle suggestions and invitations.

10   Like a broken record.

11   In the Zen Buddhist tradition, the realization of there being an awareness of non-duality is known as the 'gateless gate'. The act of perception brings potential out of consciousness into existence (matter). The act of thought brings knowledge out of mind into existence. The repetition of the latter act results in TI/ME, the content of thought. Once matter and mind have come into apparent existence, thought maintains that there has to be an inherent background to them. So it invents space for matter, and time for mind. Yet, space and time are inherently empty. Space is infinity when perceived without content, whereas time is eternity when perceived without content. Insight resides between space and infinity, and time and eternity.

12   One of the delusive aggregates which contributes to forming the notion of 'I': *ahamkara* (skt); *sanya* (pli).

13   Impression, identification, memory and experience.

14   An EEG transition from a theta brain wave state to a gamma brain wave state might provide an observable and measurable take on this, especially for those wishing to remain on the 'merrygoround' of projecting, and being validated by, a relative world. However, it is only by immersing into the felt-sense of calm intensity that insight will be born.

15   Which provides the insight of arising and passing being free from the content of thought. This insight is not the content of thought, it is its essence – the awareness of consciousness! A no 'I' perspective.

16   This take of consciousness will follow the model of: Matter to Mind to Consciousness. Rather than the model of Consciousness to Mind to Matter. The latter understanding of consciousness implies that there is a 'knowing' which is prior to the perception of thought and objects. Materialists tend to struggle with this – and they rarely get to be truly scientific about it. If they were to observe without the bias of being identified by TI/ME, it would completely open to another way of perceiving. This is a tall ask for anyone, materialist or not.

17   For example, the felt-sense of 'health' or 'light' with no opposite. Words do little justice to illustrate this, however, as they have been formulated under the premise of duality.

18   Which might be interpreted as meta awareness. Although this isn't the case as far as the understanding of how this term got coined, as the term developed from the idea that cognition could be aware of cognition. See: Flavell, J. (1979) 'Metacognition and cognitive monitoring: A new area of cognitive developmental inquiry.' *American Psychologist*, 34(10) 906. This is completely different. Cognition of cognition (metacognition) is akin to TI/ME being aware of TI/ME.

19   Or, we could use the two syllables in shimmer, 'shim' 'mer' and so on.

20   The most obvious way to get a felt-sense insight into A+P (arising and passing) is to sense it in A+P (anatomy and physiology).

21   ZPF in quantum theory is the quantum state containing no physical particles and is the energy of the 'ground' state. Also called zero-point energy. We would call this dynamic stillness or empty fullness or nothing being everything-ness.

22   Pan psychism can share some perspectives of this point of view. Yet, we are here pointing the finger at the moon (experiencing), not postulating yet another philosophy, and pan psychism is yet another philosophy, albeit one which asserts similar perspectives. It misses the major aspect which provides insight – experiencing and understanding the passing of TI/ME.

23 In Chinese philosophy, the five phases are also known as the elements (*wu ge yaosu*) consisting of earth, water, metal, fire, air.

24 The impression of permanence increases.

25 This is important to understand as the dissociation from the sense of arising is not 'passing'.

26 Enabling patterns of association which encourage explicit memory and enhancement of ventral vagal tone.

27 Enabling patterns of experience to be stored in the body/subconscious to suppress implicit memory which is perceived as overwhelming for the optimal functioning of the system. Ironically, if dorsal vagal tone becomes burdened, by this being the default tendency, then the system will result in being both overwhelmed and dysfunctional.

28 This is a very common habit observed in both over-activated and dissociated states. For more information refer to: Austin, J.H. (1999) *ZEN and the BRAIN*. London: MIT Press.

29 Calais-Germain, B. (2006) *Anatomy of Breathing*. Seattle, WA: Eastern Press.

30 Formed by the tendencies of reaction-based thought.

Chapter 5

1 While others were far more radical, maintaining that the elephants stood on a tortoise rather than a turtle!

2 See Professor Carlo Rovelli's wonderfully readable book *Seven Brief Lessons on Physics* (2016). London: Penguin, Random House. Put in a simplistic way, making it cognitively palatable for many. A good use of binary simplicity. Although it is wise to remember it is still only a finger pointing at the moon, eventually one must 'see' beyond the finger.

3 See: Taleb, N. (2013) *Antifragile*. London: Penguin Books.

4 If someone is attempting to convince you of what 'I AM' or 'No I' is, with complex philosophy, then it might be that they are disguising lack of insight with words.

5 Frequently, people espousing words which point towards non-duality hide behind their own finger (metaphorically speaking). However, END therapists, who are not so concerned with too much dialogue, tend to be much more involved with the moon (again, metaphorically speaking) itself, especially during sessions.

6 A rule of thumb.

7 To illustrate: Our senses pick up information and the brain interprets the information received. For example, the eye sense door receives light and relays the stimulus to the brain which perceives the specific input of light as an object by giving it a name and separates it from other objects.

8 As Occam concludes. However, the stagnation induced by 'simple' thought prevents insight beyond concept and duality.

9 The 'frog in the well' analogy is used to describe an individual who cannot or refuses to see the big picture because of being sheltered and close-minded by self-identified impressions of the world. It is also called 'kupamanduka' in Sanskrit (which is an old saying). For example, one has no idea what skills are required as one has been a frog in a well for the last 30 years, stuck in the same job repeating the same skills.

10 Also known as 'the stink of Zen'.

11 If there is enough awareness, which often there is due to the other practices that the student engages in.

12 Calm intensity is used to describe the seemingly paradoxical embodied amalgamation of awareness and equanimity acting as an interface to open both to dynamic stillness and TI/ME.

13 This was the underpinning philosophy of the pre-Socratic philosopher Heraclitus. *Panta rhei* – all phenomena changes and flows continuously. Notably, Heraclitus

highlights the potent nature of fire as the life-enabling force of the universe which enables an ever-transitional flux.

14 The polyvagal theory, developed by Dr Stephen Porges, offers a phylogenic model beginning with primitive survival responses and reaching the crescendo of complex social engagement responses involving a form of embodied and engaged immobilization to optimize empathic communication. See: Porges, S. (2011) 'The polyvagal theory: New insight into adaptive reactions of the autonomic nervous system.' *Cleveland Clinic Journal of Medicine,* 76(2) S86–S90.

15 See: Rosenberg, S. (2018) *The Healing Power of the Vagus Nerve: Self-Help Exercises for Anxiety, Depression, Trauma and Autism.* Berkeley, CA: North Atlantic Books.

16 However, this embodied calmness does not mean that every interaction will be like smelling roses as the sun sets. Actually, if only one person (person a) is engaged in this manner, then it is likely that this same individual will start to sense the inner world of the other person (person b), and they may sometimes not like it.

17 Which the non-dualist might find easier to appreciate than the materialist.

18 Babette Rothschild makes a distinction between empathy and compassion, empathy being the feeling with someone, and compassion being the feeling for someone.

19 Stephen Porges refers to person a in this regard as being a 'super-regulator'. I sense that the majority of people who are inspired to become a body therapist tap into this ability at some point – even if they 'forget' it, or start 'gilding the lily' with abstract rationale.

20 In this way calm intensity is a similar 'state' to that which the biodynamic craniosacral therapist calls a State of Balanced Awareness (SOBA). However, the SOBA taught in this manner is a good example of how 'simplicity' which lacks insight can become another detour for the mind to surreptitiously implement intention. In other words, if a practitioner is unaware of TI/ME passing, and understanding it as such, then TI/ME will still be ruling the roost, albeit under a different guise.

21 See: Sumner, G. and Haines, S. (2010) *Cranial Intelligence.* London: Singing Dragon.

22 It is told that Gautama (Gotoma) the Buddha instructed an experienced monk, by the name of Daruciriya, how to realize non-duality in only a few words. He said: 'In seeing, let there only be seeing. Similarly, in hearing let there only be hearing.' He continued through all of the senses, including the mind, by saying: 'In knowing, let there be mere knowing.' This is the most direct way to instruct someone to perceive TI/ME passing, without complicating it or dumbing it down.

23 Dispenza, J. (2014) *You are the Placebo: Making Your Mind Matter.* Sydney: Hay House.

24 The default mode network (DMN) of the brain is a network of interacting brain regions that are active when a person is not focused on the outside world. This network is the closest 'thing' to objectifying TI/ME itself and is measurable on an fMRI.

Chapter 6

1 Veil is used metaphorically here to imply delusion. Delusion differs from illusion in that an illusion is only a distortion of the senses, whereas delusion pertains to a distortion of mental perception.

2 'City' is the term used to convey the potency, magnitude and far-reaching impact of embodying this quality. In sankhya philosophy, the Sanskrit word for 'city' is used as a metaphor to stand for pure consciousness.

3 One who dwells in the 'city', in sankhya philosophy, is a metaphor used to describe someone aware of their original nature (*purusha*).

4 The simplified version of calm in-10-city is the four chambers of non-doing.

5 *Li* in this context is the Chinese word (pin yin) meaning 'organic patterns'. Jason Gregory translates this word beautifully in his book (Gregory, J. (2018) *Effortless Living.* Rochester, VT: Inner Traditions/Bear).

6   www.dhamma.org.

7   This does not mean that intentional imagination is taboo; it can be useful to prime the ability to sense passing. For example, when a practitioner 'widens' their perceptual field of awareness by imagining their mind being out as far as the wall limits of the room they are in, or if needed as far as the limits of the town, country or universe, then the reality of space gets a chance to present itself. The important thing to remember with this is to sense the passing nature of the imagination and let the reality of space awareness remain in its wake. Such awareness will now be vibrant, whole and unhindered by stealth intention(s).

8   www.bodyintelligence.com. Also see: *Cranial Intelligence* by Ged Sumner and Steve Haines (2010). London: Singing Dragon.

Chapter 7

1   Or, the dissociated from experience mind.

2   In the context of where it fits in to enhancing access attention, SOBA and calm intensity.

3   These limbs are: *yama* (morality discipline), *niyama* (self-discipline), *asana* (steady, comfortable postures), *pran-ayama* (awareness of the natural breath), *pratyahara* (internalization), *dharana* (sustained attention), *dhyana* (meditation), *samadhi* (liberation).

4   Sanskrit: *ahimsa*.

5   Patanjali is said to have stated that *yama, niyama, asana, pran-ayama, pratyahara, dharana, dhyana* and *samadhi* are the ingredients needed to be liberated. However, Patanjali then notes that after starting this process, the blockage to liberation is *yama, niyama, pran-ayama, pratyahara, dharana, dhyana* and *samadhi*. In other words, right intention sets the course for liberation but intention needs to pass for liberation to occur.

6   Calming curl (spinal flexion).

7   And bionimbus (aura).

8   In *dharana trataka* practice this method is known as *shamb-havi mudra*.

9   In *dharana trataka* practice this method is known as *nasika-gra*.

10 SASA is used here as a tongue in cheek imitation of NASA to highlight the launching of a journey into the universe of non-doing.

11 This is useful to open to the gut space, and thereby open to the spaces of the body in general. This is the *tan-tien* and lower and deep to this is the *swadhisthana* chakra.

12 *Manipura* chakra.

13 This is known in Sanskrit as *daharakasha*; an appreciation of the origins of this area. An amalgamation of *mooladhara, swadhisthana* and *manipura* chakras.

14 In Sanskrit, the perception of the heart space is known as *hri-dayakasha*.

15 Mistaken by some as control of the breath. Actually it is awareness of the uncontrolled breath *pran-ayama*.

16 The space of the cranium is known in Sanskrit as *chidakasha*.

17 This scooping and funnelling is called the Flehmen response and is only activated in certain mammals even though humans can voluntarily curl the upper lip up into exactly the same position as, say, a horse.

18 This is breath-work, not *pran-ayama*.

19 Breath-fast is now effortless.

20 See: McKeown, P. (2015) *The Oxygen Advantage*. New York, NY: William Morrow Publishing.

21 Attention is the stretching of awareness.

22 Understanding (*jnana/nana*) of the arising and passing of sensations.

23 Cranio-spinal cavity, deriving from ectoderm, containing four brain chambers: two lateral ventricles, third ventricle and fourth ventricle. Thoracic cavity, deriving from mesoderm, containing four heart chambers: two atriums and two ventricles. Abdominal cavity (including esophagus), deriving from endoderm containing four gut chambers: esophagus, stomach, small intestine and large intestine.

24 Calm intensity is the gateless gate to dynamic stillness.

Chapter 8

1 Ground intent is the becoming from the universal rather than becoming from the conditioned/particular.

2 The dissolution of the objectified impression of that to reveal 'its' essential nature.

3 The ease: exploration, expansion, expression, ephemerality and emptiness.

4 See: Gilder, L. (2009) *The Age of Entanglement: When Quantum Physics Was Reborn.* New York, NY: Vintage Publications.

5 Insight expands our ability to sense subtlety and realize the intimate connection to our infinite environment. This could be regarded as 'knowing' rather than 'known'.

6 Term inspired by talks given by Jean Klein, Francis Lucille and Rupert Spira.

7 Materialists come from a 'practical' perspective which bases itself on a primary matter = mind = consciousness model, whereas this 'model' (if it is reduced to being called a model) bases itself on the premise that consciousness = mind = matter, from a wholistic perspective, i.e. the other way around; and matter = mind = consciousness from a relative perspective. But the model is only a vicious cycle for the mind until the felt-sense reality moves one beyond TI/ME's limits. So, from a relative perspective, 'fragmented consciousness' is the processing and negotiation of the brain in response to the body's encounters and movement. However, it can be argued that fragmented consciousness is not consciousness in and of itself, as the 'hard problem of consciousness' would attest. Here is an analogy to illustrate: fragmented consciousness is akin to the whirlpools and eddy currents formed in a stream (the stream being a metaphor for 'primary consciousness'). The seemingly individual currents form 'relative consciousness', and perceive/identify themselves as divided movements (objects) separate from each other and the stream. However, the flow of the stream is a divisionless movement, and insight dawns when fragmented consciousness (TI/ME) is also perceived as divisionless (i.e. arising and passing, not being separate – a divisionless vibration). When an individual maintains that cognition equates to consciousness they are, it is hoped, talking about the body shaping the brain to form the mind (TI/ME), to then produce thought. Yet, as has been proposed throughout this book, thought is manifested and propelled by both TI/ME and insight. Remember, insight, in this context, is the awareness of TI/ME passing and the felt-sense of arising and passing (non-separate, same). The intimate vibration of arising and passing (consciousness) is present before, during and after the seeming display of TI/ME.

8 Rather than solidifying potential 'things' into existence via a conditioned narrative (accumulation of TI/ME). See articles on the delayed choice experiments: Kaiser, F., Coudreau, T., Milman, P. and Ostrowsky, D.B. (2012) 'Entanglement-enabled delayed choice experiment.' *Science, 338*(6107) 637–640; Peruzzo, A., Shadbolt, P., Brunne, N., Popescu, S. and O'Brien, J.L. (2012) 'A quantum delayed-choice experiment.' *Science, 338*(6107) 634–637. We cloister freedom with TI/ME and 'it' becomes jolly practical – until jolly is seen for what it really is!

9 See: Spira, R. (2017) *Being Aware of Being Aware.* Oxford: Sahaja Publications.

10 Not experience, which is part of TI/ME.

11 See: Frydman, M. and Dikshit, S.S. (2008) *I Am That. Talks with Sri Nisar-gadatta Maharaj.* Durham, NC: The Acorn Press.

12   Please note that this is not a form of 'distance healing'. Rather, it is realizing the reactive tendencies within oneself which helps to settle all that we are subtly in contact with. This is as far as this insight needs to go from an intellectual understanding standpoint. If we start to think we are 'healing' another when such settling takes place then we are surreptitiously setting up yet another reactive tendency leading to another subtle intention.

13   Gabor Maté: Hungarian-born Canadian physician specializing in helping addiction and trauma. Bestselling author of many books including *In the Realm of Hungry Ghosts* (2009). London: Random House. The account shared by Dr Maté was during the 2020 online Embodiment conference.

14   The acronym SPEND is used here to illustrate the way that the insight of TI/ME passing, acknowledged by the therapist, is being spent on opening to the expression of health in the client. In this context, insight is inexhaustible, the same way that the sun shines without needing to refuel. 'This' is TI/ME well spent!

15   Each individual will be able to access and 'augment' the subtle awareness of their major senses with differing success. Some might have a powerful predisposition to resonate with the subtlety of vision consciousness. This can result in the balance point being perceived as white light, which is a potent awareness of the third ventricle. Others might have a subtle awareness of auditory consciousness; this is often perceived as an unlabellable sound, which can at times seem like sound originating from outside but is in fact a deep and potent tone from within the third ventricle. It is good here to discover whether you have a propensity to one of the sense consciousness vibrations. If, after some time of checking out the subtle light or sound it becomes apparent that the sense consciousness is not developed in you, then it is useful to develop the touch awareness of an isolated area of the body first. It can take an extremely long time to develop the subtle awareness of vision and auditory consciousness. The awareness of sensations arising and passing on one area of the body is perfectly sufficient for opening to calm intensity, so don't get side-tracked. A point of caution for those who do have a propensity to open to the third ventricle: If you establish a one-pointed attention here (cittass-ekaggata) then remember not to get stuck as if the body does not exist. Such a state serves no purpose as a body therapist. When you include the now subtle and potent awareness of your body then you will be treating from a very equanimous calm intensity and the client's body will feel met and safe to express at sometimes great depth.

16   See: www.betterearthing.com.au.

Chapter 9

1   This is very different from disassociation from TI/ME; dissociation is TI/ME itself catalysing distraction, whereas disassociation from TI/ME is awareness being aware of the passing of TI/ME.

2   In other words it is a choice. Awareness, in the deepest sense of that word, is not a choice – awareness is. J. Krishnamurti calls such awareness 'choiceless'.

3   Dissociation out of awareness is the ultimate duality, therefore the deepest cause of anguish, despite the possibility of perceiving a sense of 'oneness'. This is because TI/ME now projects the impression of an alternative experience, seemingly free from suffering and entranced by pleasure.

4   He used the word impermanence rather than TI/ME passing.

5   Shakespeare phrase pointing at how the mind projects 'good' onto an experience.

6   Zen saying, pointing at how the mind projects 'bad' onto an experience.

Chapter 10

1   The non-doing felt-sense of increased attunement. Touch here being an excuse for the client to feel tangibly met (somatically heard) as we listen to the biodynamic expressions of their system, while acknowledging our own original nature.

2   'Hard materialists' do not accept that a person's felt-sense is anything more than a mental interpretation of a physical world. In other words their understanding of consciousness is nothing more than it being brain activity.

'Soft materialists' do not accept that all felt-sense perceptions are physical ones. They concede, hopefully via insight, that consciousness is more than just a brain processing the body's encounters and negotiating the world.

The mind and body are related and do not act independently of each other, but the mind is informed by more than just the body. Whereas some idealists tend to go to the other extreme and promote the idea of the mind being solely formed from consciousness, which is true if matter is also conscious...but their premise is usually by way of belief rather than insight.

Insight of TI/ME passing is akin to a light shining and illuminating how we get blinkered into thinking the accrual of conditioned reactions are the reason for consciousness, while concurrently realizing the shining light itself is consciousness.

3   Materialists offer a sane, rational, logical argument for the way we perceive the world. The formation and shaping of the mind occurs due to the body's movement and interactions with the world. A bottom-up effect rather than a top-down effect.

Yet, unfortunately, materialists (especially hard materialists) very rarely concede their premise sufficiently to access the felt-sense intimacy needed to answer the 'hard question', such as 'what is consciousness itself?' Without answering this, in a grounded manner, all meaningful questions (i.e. those which acknowledge human dis-satisfactoriness) which open to a perception which is not merely temporarily satisfying, remain unanswered!

By discarding potential felt-sense insight, of TI/ME passing, in favour of interpreting matter as the sole reason for consciousness, is like throwing the baby out with the bath water and getting fixated with the image of the bath!

4   This is a tongue-in-cheek comment, but hopefully it illustrates how we can get caught into doing despite thinking we are non-doing.

5   Materialist:

Matter ➡ Mind ⟶ Consciousness

What is consciousness in this regard? Consciousness here is the outcome following the interpretation of sense derived phenomena. So, the interpretation of phenomena, by a seemingly separate self, results in TI/ME, which is then regarded as consciousness...i.e. 'me' being conscious despite it being an impression of matter.

Idealist:

Consciousness ➡ Mind ⟶ Matter

What is consciousness in this regard? Consciousness here is an eternal omni-present and omnipotent force/intelligence, such as God, limiting itself by projecting the world, through TI/ME, providing an impression of the phenomenal world.

END therapist:

Dynamic stillness ★ Calm intensity (insight mind) ★ Matter

What is consciousness in this regard? It is 'This'...When the arrows disappear (i.e. no more model) dynamic stillness, calm intensity and matter are all consciousness.

Key:

➡ Absolute

⟶ Impression

★ Felt-sense awareness of arising and passing freeing itself from the limitation of being perceived as a model.

6   The Buddhist *Mahasatipatthana Sutta* emphasises the importance of becoming familiar with the sensations within the sensations.

7   Specifically the *Visudhimagga* (Path of purification).

8   Important Buddhist commentary compiled in Sri Lanka during the fifth century AD.

9   See: Wallace, B.A. (2010) *Distorted Visions of Buddhism: Agnostic and Atheist.* New York, NY: Spiegel & Grau.

10   In addition to many well-known people such as Aldous Huxley, David Bohm, Greta Garbo and Charlie Chaplin.

11   Professor David Bohm was an eminent scientist noted by Albert Einstein to be the person to take his reins.

12   Including the lack of felt-sense connection due to lack of early secure attachment.

13   See: Schore, A.N. (1994) *Affect Regulation and the Origin of the Self*. Hillsdale, NJ: Lawrence Erlbaum Associates.

14   Which prevents the felt-sense of 'independent integration'. An ethological example: A baby elephant will need to be guided by its mother and troop or it will likely become prey to potential dangers. However, when it has orientated to the environment, it becomes 'independently integrated'. This was evident when a huge tsunami hit Sri Lanka in 2004. Hours prior to the wave hitting shore, while people were still unaware and resting on the beach, the elephant troops all headed inland en mass. (See: *National Geographic*, 4 January 2005). It was later reported that prior to the tsunami, dogs refused to go outdoors, flamingos abandoned their low-lying breeding areas and zoo animals rushed to their shelters and could not be enticed out. Thousands of people perished during this same tsunami along India's Cuddalore coast, yet buffalos, goats and dogs were found unharmed.

15   J. Krishnamurti considers the realization and felt-sense contact with our original nature, in day-to-day life, as relationship itself.

16   Which the brain stimulating attachment first put us in contact with.

17   And to a degree the sense of taste via mouth-breathing.

18   Such as *Conscious* by Annaka Harris. Annaka's book is a very palatable read, for most people, and helps calm the mind down by sanely informing the reader of how matter shapes consciousness. She takes the subject far enough to touch the border of the materialist's perspective of consciousness. When the mind has become balanced from this vantage point we can delve deeper. See: Harris, A. (2019) *Conscious*. New York, NY: HarperCollins.

   J. Krishnamurti often spoke about the importance of putting the 'house of the mind' in order before inquiring into the deep issues, such as meditation (inquiry into the passing of TI/ME). This book provides a good resource for achieving this.

19   www.hooponopono.org.

20   Once you realize 'This' there is an act of potentially beholding it everywhere. It is interesting to note that the etymologic derivation of the word 'This' comes from the act of beholding, rather than from perceiving or identifying with a particular object. So 'This' (with a capital T) is another word for awareness of awareness being aware.

21   With felt-sense awareness of TI/ME passing one will eventually, insightfully, realize that the observer is the observed. This cannot be understood philosophically.

22   Inspired by Rupert Spira: www.rupertspira.com.

23   At the time of writing this book, Rupert was in the process of publishing the 'I Am' poem in a new book (*A meditation on; I am*, see references). I encourage you to acquire this book, as the poem is very inspiring and insightfully articulated.

24   The Fawn response is a term coined by Pete Walker MA, MFT to describe the inherent defence response used to placate outer conflict and suppress internal conflict. See www.pete-walker.com and his (2015) book *The Tao of Fully Feeling*. Lafayette, CA: Azure Coyote Publishing. Pete Walker also describes how this response can be combined with other psychologic survival responses (e.g. fawn-fight/passive-aggressive) to form a hybrid defence strategy.

25   Surrender to another's overt or covert demands with enough cognitive ability to understand that to do otherwise would lead to danger.

26   It is the understanding of this reality which guided some people to retreat from the distractions of worldly affairs to realize the subtle inner world of TI/ME arising/passing, eventuating, at some point, with the end of dis-satisfactoriness. Nevertheless, this is only half the journey, the second half is re-entering the world of duality with

the insight of non-duality and helping others to co-regulate, without dependence, to help enhance potential moments of insight.

Despite this, a great many recluses remain in the comfort of the first half of the journey without insight, which is a real pity, as this becomes yet another technique offering freedom, but is merely decorating a prison cell. The delusion of such illusory freedom dissolves when one wakes to the relational field of TI/ME arising and passing, which is where real freedom resides.

27 Felt-sense awareness of body weight (e.g. one leg compared to the other), the outline of their body, skin awareness and their inner felt-sense.

Chapter 11

1 Relaxes due to trusting, rather than dissociating through fear.

2 Leather glove used for training birds of prey.

3 Especially when it also knows it will be fed.

4 There is a fair amount of evidence to suggest that a majority of people would prefer to feel acute discomfort rather than feel nothing. In the research studies, it is not clear whether the 'nothing' referred to is dissociation from sensations or opening to the unfamiliar. I suspect it is the latter.

5 From seeming to be a jigsaw puzzle of fragments to a more whole body sense.

6 In fact, the END therapist will be providing a sense of engaged safety which is likely to remind the subconscious of a figure from the past who gave them adequate resource for their body to express health.

Chapter 12

1 For example, holding an uncomfortable posture for a set period of time helps the mindset to become familiar with relative discomfort, knowing that it will pass. The insight of this event deepens as one becomes aware of TI/ME passing during the posture. This is the very vitality people often feel during yoga classes.

2 The word *pran-ayama* is really two Sanskrit words: *prana* and *ayama*. This is often misunderstood and many students think the two words are *prana* and *yama*. *Yama* means to restrain or control, *ayama* means not to do that.

Excerpt from a book by Bernie Clarke called *Yin Yoga, the Philosophy & Practice of Yin Yoga*. See references.

3 Patanjali is said to have stated that *yama, niyama, asana, pran-ayama, pratyahara, dharana, dhyana* and *samadhi* are the ingredients needed to be liberated. However, Patanjali then notes that after starting this process the blockage to liberation is *yama, niyama, pran-ayama, pratyahara, dharana, dhyana* and *samadhi*. In other words, right intention sets the course for liberation but intention needs to pass for it to be so.

4 This could also be called the 'orientation response' if the setting is mostly perceived as being safe already. The term 'apprehension reflex' was borrowed from my friend Kit Laughlin, who used it in the context of describing the acknowledgment of apprehension and the utilisation of this awareness to recruit techniques which provide the felt sense of safety to counter potential restrictions in one's flexibility. The first use of the term, 'Apprehension Reflex (AR)', was in his book *Overcome Neck & Back Pain, 4th edition* (2016, p.35).

This is the third reflex in Kit's Stretch Therapy approach. The term describes the increased capacity to stretch if the person stretching has one part of their body limiting further stretching of one of the joints involved in the movement. For example, a standard stretch for the hamstrings is to bend forward over straight legs. Kit found that if the person stretching places a rolled mat between trunk and thighs – so the brain can feel the position of the thighs in relation to the body – usable flexibility increases immediately. On being questioned, students reply that the position 'feels safer' and their apprehension has reduced. For example, they feel that the tension in the muscles has reduced, and that they can stretch further as a result.

5   Some may consider this meditation. It may be more appropriate to consider this the foundation for insight to unfold, which could then lead to meditation.

6   A term Stanley Rosenberg uses in his wonderful book: *Accessing the Healing Power of the Vagus Nerve* (see references).

7   The 'Fold response' is the term used to describe how the autonomic nervous system responds to threat by inducing hypotonic dissociation.
    Survival 'F' responses include: Friend, Fond, Fight, Flight, Freeze, Fold/Fawn, Fairies.

8   *Agochari mudra*, the gesture of looking at the nose tip (calming) and shambhavi mudra, the gesture of looking up at the area between the eyebrows (energising) are two examples.

9   Name for this gentle stimulation in Sanskrit is *balayam*. Some yogis maintain that this stimulation promotes hair growth.

10 Indian sage thought to have lived during the 2nd century BC. There is doubt whether one sole character was the author of what was said to be written by him (the yoga sutras). Nevertheless, he (or she) was certainly very influential to the development of ancient yoga practice.

11 For more information, see Kit Laughlin's book *Stretching & Flexibility* in references.

12 See Kotler, S. (2015) *The Rise of Superman. Decoding the Science of Ultimate Human Performance*. London: Quercus Books.

13 Which is insensitivity of the body and a deep identification with TI/ME (ignorance).

14 With relevant mechanical intention.

Chapter 13

1   In Chinese, there is a similar word called *jen* (*zhun*) introduced and promoted by the infamous philosopher Confucius.

2   Bohannon, J. (2014) 'Electric shock study suggests we'd rather hurt ourselves than others'. www.sciencemag.org.

3   See: Miller, D.T. (1999) 'The norm of self interest.' *American Psychology, 54*: 1053–1060.

4   See: Piff, P.K., Stancato, D.M., Cote, S., Mendoza-Denton, R. and Keltner, D. (2012) 'Higher social class predicts increased unethical behaviour.' *Proceedings of the National Academy of Sciences,* 109(11) 4086–4091.

5   Crockett, M.J., Kurth-Nelson, Z., Siegle, J.Z., Dayan, P. and Dolan, R.J. (2014) 'Harm to others outweighs harm to self in moral decision making.' *Proceedings of the National Academy of Sciences,* 111(48) 17320–17325.

6   The next step, Crockett says, is to do the experiments while scanning people's brains to 'investigate how these [moral] computations go awry in disorders like psychopathy'. 'This is a landmark study,' says Johannes Haushofer, a psychologist at Princeton University. The result is 'both obvious and surprising'. Intuition dictates that people should be willing to give up some money to avoid the distress of hurting someone. But 'despite decades of research, the effect had not previously been demonstrated', he says. It may be possible to tap into this altruism simply by reminding people in positions of power – from chefs to politicians – of the painful consequences of their decisions to cut corners.

7   See: Crocker, J., Canevello, A. and Brown, A. (2016) 'Social motivation costs and benefits of selfishness and otherishness.' *Annual Review of Psychology, 68*: 299–325.

Glossary

1   *Li* in this context is the Chinese word (pin yin) meaning 'organic pattern'.

Index